SOCIOLOGY AND HEALTH

This lively, introductory text provides students and health practitioners with the foundations of a sociological understanding of health issues. Written for anyone who is interested in health and disease in contemporary global society, this book engages the reader to act upon their occupational and moral responsibilities.

It explains the key sociological theories and debates with humour and imagination in a way that will encourage an inquisitive and reflective approach on the part of any student who engages with the text. With individual chapters covering sociology, health, science, power, medicalisation, madness, happiness, sex, violence, and death, *Sociology and Health* is organised so that the student moves through sociological approaches and themes which constantly recur in the experience of healthcare.

Students will find this a readable and controversial text which covers the ground they need to know in a thought-provoking way. Lecturers will find it a helpful text for generating discussion in tutorials and seminars. There are summaries at the end of each chapter, suggestions for further reading, and ideas for the reader.

Peter Morrall is Senior Lecturer in Health and Sociology at the University of Leeds, UK.

SOCIOLOGY AND HEALTH

AN INTRODUCTION

Second edition

PETER MORRALL

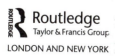

Routledge
Taylor & Francis Group

LONDON AND NEW YORK

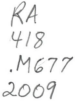

First published 2001

This edition published 2009
by Routledge
2 Park Square, Milton Park, Abingdon, Oxon OX14 4RN

Simultaneously published in the USA and Canada
by Routledge
270 Madison Avenue, New York, NY 10016

Routledge is an imprint of the Taylor & Francis Group,
an informa business

© 2001, 2009 Peter Morrall

Typeset in Times New Roman and Futura by
Florence Production, Stoodleigh, Devon
Printed and bound in Great Britain by
CPI, Antony Rowe, Chippenham, Wiltshire

British Library Cataloguing in Publication Data
A catalogue record for this book is available from the British Library

Library of Congress Cataloging-in-Publication Data
Morrall, Peter.
  Sociology and health: an introduction/
Peter Morrall.
      p. cm.
  Rev. ed. of: Sociology and nursing/Peter Morrall. 2001.
    Includes bibliographical references and index.
  1. Social medicine.   2. Sociology.   3. Nursing – Social
aspects.   I. Morrall, Peter. Sociology and nursing.   II. Title.
  RA418.M677 2009
  362.1—dc22   2008038199

ISBN10: 0–415–41562–4 (hbk)
ISBN10: 0–415–41563–2 (pbk)
ISBN10: 0–203–88132–X (ebk)

ISBN13: 978–0–415–41562–0 (hbk)
ISBN13: 978–0–415–41563–7 (pbk)
ISBN13: 978–0–203–88132–3 (ebk)

All it takes for evil to triumph in the world is
for good men [and women] to do nothing.

(Edmond Burke – allegedly)

CONTENTS

ABBREVIATIONS

AAAS	American Association for the Advancement of Science
CAM	complementary-alternative medicine
CPN	community psychiatric nurse
DHHS	Department of Health and Human Services
DOA	dead on arrival
ESRC	Economic and Social Research Council
MRSA	methicillin-resistant staphylococcus aureus
NHS	National Health Service
PTSD	post-traumatic stress disorder
RCT	randomised-control trial
SSRI	selective serotonin re-uptake inhibitor
WHO	World Health Organization

INTRODUCTION

'M ANGRY, AS ANGRY AS HELL. What's my anger about? Here's a hint:

> Globally, there are more than 1 billion overweight adults, at least 300 million of them obese. Obesity and overweight pose a major risk for chronic diseases, including type 2 diabetes, cardiovascular disease, hypertension and stroke, and certain forms of cancer. The key causes are increased consumption of energy-dense foods high in saturated fats and sugars, and reduced physical activity.
>
> (World Health Organization, 2008a)

> Every day, on average, more than 26,000 children under age five die around the world, mostly from preventable causes.
>
> (United Nations Children's Fund, 2008: 6)

MESS

My good friend and spiritual antagonist (a certain Reverend Alan Brown), a man I admire for his tenacious attempts over many years to convert me to his faith (or any faith), has a wonderful expression when trying to placate my agitation (about so many things): 'Well, Peter, it's a messy world'. Indeed, the world is in a mess. It's always been in a mess, but humans have somehow managed to muddle through the mire of their own making. Those who have tried to tidy up (the Romans, Crusaders, Mongols, Islamists, Nazis, neoconservatives) have generally caused more mess in their attempts or wake than was there in the first place. However, human societies and the physical environment have adapted and persisted. But muddling through the present mess could be impossible. We may well be doomed, and it might be time to panic.

Social and health inequalities are worsening. While the majority of people in the world struggle with poverty and disease, and die at an early age, a minority is getting richer, becoming less diseased, living much longer, but paradoxically are not much happier. Moreover, the natural world upon which human health is so dependent is tipping towards catastrophic collapse and in the process generating more poverty and disease, and civilisation itself is threatened (Brown, 2008; World Wildlife Fund, 2008). The impending ecological death of the earth, of course, is the ultimate health problem for humanity.

We all know about the mess. It is broadcast constantly on our television screens, written about regularly in our newspapers; it is the plot of successful documentary films, and there is an abundance of literature in our high streets and Internet bookstores on its every aspect. Moreover, the majority of people in the world are acutely aware that the world is messy because they live *in* a mess. For them, dealing with food crises, seeking clean water, and not succumbing to sickness *is* their life.

So, what is the common reaction from those of us who (as yet) are not forced to exist in the bowels of global society, given that the media's proctoscopic gaze provides such detailed imagery, exhaustive diagnosis, and terminal prognosis about the state of the world?: disinterest, disillusionment, and diversion! Sociologists Stan Cohen and Laurie Taylor (1992) point out that those in Westernised societies spend much of their lives indulging in 'escape attempts' to avoid not only the realities of others' lives but also the meaninglessness and awfulness of their own existence. We switch off our consciousness and conscience about the mess and deal with the minutiae of our daily routines, soothing our souls and numbing our minds with a soap opera, sun-drenched holiday, shuffle around the shops, or frothy coffees and fat-laden food. We bury our humane emotions and human intellect until unpreventable death while others bury their loved ones who have died too young from preventable deaths.

This book is an introduction to sociological thinking about a major component of messy human reality – health. However, there are many such books. Indeed, this one is a follow-up from my own sociological critique of nursing (Morrall, 2001). The target readership is primarily anyone working in or studying the field, but a subsidiary target readership is those who already have (perhaps considerable) knowledge about the sociology of health.

My intention is to inform but also to be uncompromisingly and unapologetically provocative. The provocation is directed towards those who have been the target of critique by sociologists (particularly doctors and nurses) *and* those who have provided the critique (that is, sociological establishment) – a plague on both houses (or at least some of the rooms within them).

MORALITY

The brief here is to present key ideas about health in the context of *global* society to the main occupational groups working in health including managers, bureaucrats, and politicians (as well as those who study the subject: for example, sociologists, anthropologists, and human geographers). The hard-hitting message is: health is an ethical issue. That is, medical and health practitioners (together with social scientists) not only have occupational responsibilities but a *moral* responsibility for health.

Moreover, in a globalised society this responsibility extends beyond local health to *global* health. It is morally inexcusable to be constrained by one's career, to care only for those suffering from the indulgencies of a consumer culture, for the cosmetically challenged, or the self-centredly sad, while children and adults rot and expire unnecessarily within *their* global society. Such abrogation of moral responsibility is akin to doctors and nurses leaving two-thirds of their patients on a hospital ward to writhe in excruciating pain or slowly starve to death while they attentively care for the other third (who just happen to be private patients). But it is not a few on a ward that are being seriously neglected but a billion in the world (Collier, 2007).

The 'wider picture' not only needs to be understood by medical and health practitioners (which has been offered to them by sociologists for decades) but their role in the treatment of this messy world must become part of their occupational obligation (a new demand made by this sociologist). The dynamic role of sociology in comprehending human health is well established. That society induces health and disease is incontrovertible. William Cockerham, Professor of Sociology at the University of Alabama at Birmingham, puts it thus:

> It is clear that most diseases have social connotations. That is, the social context can shape the risk of exposure, the susceptibility of the host, and the disease's course and outcome – regardless of whether the disease is infectious, genetic, metabolic, malignant, or degenerative.

(Cockerham, 2007: 2)

The public recognise that social factors can make them either more or less healthy. Medical and health practitioners are taught sociology in their basic training and adopt sociological concepts in their academic literature. Politicians in departments of health instigate research and policies that include sociological investigative tools and sociologically informed recommendations. The bureaucrats, who have invaded both state and private health systems, may even have been introduced to the ideas of Karl Marx on their MBA courses.

However, although social factors are realised, reality doesn't change correspondingly. Sociology demystifies the nature of health and illness, highlights the social causes of disease and death, exposes power factors and ethical dilemmas in the production of healthcare, and either directly or indirectly helps to create a discerning practitioner who then becomes capable of more focused and competent decision making.

However, the world remains a mess.

I do not wish to overstate the case for sociology. The contribution of sociology must not be at the expense of practical skills and direct knowledge of human physiology and pathology needed by medical and health practitioners. It must certainly not be at the expense of cleanliness, kindliness, and clinical competence. Furthermore, this is an era of revolutionary ('hard') science and technology. Starting in the latter part of the twentieth century, unprecedented discoveries and the reshaping of human knowledge about the physical world has taken place. In the fields of physics, chemistry, mathematics, computing, pharmacology, genetics, and medicine, the accumulation of and transformation in knowledge has been nothing short of incredible.

Moreover, many sociologists are also disinterested, disillusioned, and diverted. Their disinterest is apparent by the lack of genuine activism emanating from the discipline and the loss of radical intellectualism (Furedi, 2004). Their disillusionment is understandable because the universities have become mass-education assembly lines disgorging a contagion of puerile 'outcomes' and pathetic 'skills', thereby 'killing thinking' (Evans, 2005). Their digression is exemplified in the mental-masturbatory socio-twaddle[1] of postmodernist posturing by 'intellectual impostures' (Sokal and Bricmont, 2003). The routing of sexual energy into genital-auto-stimulation is normal and healthy. The routing of academic energy into the nihilistic futility of resolute deconstructionism (the conjecture that *nothing* is real to anyone) and cerebral sludge of cultural relativism (the conjecture that *anything* can be real to someone) is dissolute and damned dangerous when human suffering on such a scale is at stake. To wilfully mix metaphors: sociology 'lost the plot' at the 'postmodern turn'.

POSITION

Positions taken by anyone on any subject are reached as a consequence of the interplay between personal and prescribed considerations. My stance on sociology and health has been seeded by the reflexive entwining of learning from living (encounters, events, and cultures) and learning about life (formal study). Therefore, both require detailing to appreciate that stance. This is not a matter of self-indulgence, but an essential exposure of my personal background and academic foreground to allow the reader to judge how justified I am in taking the stance I do on sociology and health.

I was brought up in a violent and impoverished slum area in the north of England, which, although in the mid-twentieth century, resembled Frederick Engels' (1845) lurid account of the living conditions of the working class from more than a hundred years previously. Since then I have witnessed first-hand the dying and death of young and old people from ferocious and foul cancers, and from both speedily terminal and cruelly prolonged heart diseases. I have got to know well scores of people of various ages with degenerative neurological disorders that long before death result in sentient minds being trapped in and tortured by disobedient and disintegrating bodies, and those who (perhaps more fortunately) have succumbed to the reverse of this mind–body split.

Incarcerated within 'colonies' for 'subnormals', I have come across people with life-defying mental and physical handicaps, adolescents with bone-breaking and face-disfiguring epilepsy, and children with such grossly self-injurious behaviour that they either had to be drugged into passivity or wrapped in straitjackets and placed in padded cells. These repositories for human imperfection also contained idiot savants. These people could not do the most basic of tasks such as feed or dress themselves but might have one complex skill such as playing the piano by ear or remembering thousands of car number plates along with the names of the relevant owners.

Through a long association with madness, and more recently with murder, working in or for asylums, prisons, and special institutions for the criminally insane, I've come to know much about human munificence and human malevolence. There have been some interesting and disturbing characters along the way: a necrophiliac (who really did have the job of his dreams working in a mortuary); two Jesus Christs (who were engaged in a rather unchristian prolonged dispute over which of them was the real Messiah until they were becalmed by antipsychotic medication); and a multitude of people diagnosed as 'psychopathic' (some of whom craved attention while others craved killing).

Long before cheap mass tourism took off, I travelled around the world. Through travel I have met with a kaleidoscope of peoples and cultures. I've been horrified by emaciated and decomposing bodies of the dispossessed on busy third-world streets and dismayed at the plight of fly-covered pot-bellied children, exasperated by the flatulent views and incontinent behaviours of the nouveau riche, and puzzled over what the emotional pay-off is for the super-rich from their compulsion to accumulate and conspicuously exhibit their wealth. I have slept in doorways, ditches, and deserts, as well as in deluxe hotels, ridden a motorcycle through a riot and been party to the kidnapping of a policeman by a bunch of hippies on a bus during a revolution.

My education in sociology began in 1980 and continues to intrigue me, as do my excursions into criminology and psychology and tentative forays into natural science. At first I was seduced (willingly) by the sages of sociology. Then, similar to the emotional despair from discovering that an idealised lover is an unfaithful fake, I became deeply saddened by the pathetic pretentiousness and naivety of those purporting to be scholars of society. I now have far more respect for those whose role is to have direct day-to-day responsibility for, or research into, the suffering of others than I have for those who recklessly deconstruct those roles and the suffering, having themselves no more responsibility than finishing their next unfathomable tract for delivery at an unattended seminar or submission to an unread journal.

What I regard as the vital strength of sociology is its scepticism. Sociology, through scepticism, has profound insights and directions to offer the field of human health. Sociology has also to be sceptical about its own constructions. For example, my ideas continue to mature and modify, and I am aware of my own cognitive limitations and perceptual parameters. I'm no stranger to being in the wrong.

However, scepticism is not cynicism. Refusing to take anything at 'face value' is not a recommendation to 'value nothing'. Challenging constructions within the field of health must lead to reconstruction not destruction. Destructiveness by the mental masturbators of sociology is as immoral as 'asocial' medicine and nursing (or any occupation dealing with human health).

Moreover, the intellectual insularity of these occupations is exacerbated by the contemporary crusade for 'evidence-based practice' founded on a specific and disputable type of science (empiricism). Empirical evangelism, whether preached by social or natural scientists, is pretentious and naive, and, like mental masturbation, also damned dangerous. An inflamed importance given to empirical data ('empiricalitis'), whether spawned from quantitative or qualitative research, overlooks or underplays social contexts that always have some degree of influence on human performance[2], including health. Alternative modes of explanation such as intuition, inspiration, argument, artistry, or custom, are ignored, ridiculed, or, if too much of a threat, colonised. The notion that as yet unknown ways of understanding the social and natural worlds (epistemologies other than that of empiricism) is unrecognised or discounted.

Cecil Helman, general practitioner, psychiatrist, social anthropologist, and publisher of the acclaimed text 'Culture, Health and Illness', believes that medicine is an art as well as a science, and about uncertainty as much as certainty. This is contrary to what he was taught during his initial medical training:

> At medical school, in our textbooks and lectures, diseases were described to us as if they were abstract 'things', somehow independent of the people who suffered from them. And independent, too, of their religious or social backgrounds, or the particular and unique circumstances of their personal lives, such as stress, unhappiness, poverty, discrimination, or poor housing. Most importantly, this approach left out the *meanings* that people give to their illnesses. . . . It left out, too, all of the stories they tell . . . endless cycles of stories, whether poetic or banal, many hidden within other stories, or concealed behind the masks of symptoms or disease.
>
> (Helman, 2006: 7–8; emphasis in the original)

Recently retired from family practice after nearly three decades, Helman is worried that improvements in medical appreciation of social factors, global trends, cultural variations, and personal narratives is being displaced because of the requisites of 'techno-doctoring'. For Helman an over-reliance on science is short-sighted.

But this is an understatement of the problem. The blind (postmodern sociologists) are leading the blind (empirical evangelists), clinging to each other like two sightless sumo wrestlers both desperate to win but unable to release the other as either may then stumble and so lose the contest. What neither can see is the blindingly obvious: the game has become inconsequential because the audience (health consumers and disease sufferers) has come to believe that the game is fixed or irrelevant.

So, my life's experiences (so far), *reflexively* integrated with the imagination of sociology, have made me sceptical but above all a *realist*. A damned *angry* realist!

My realism with reference to health is the equivalent to that of Professor Jock Young's in criminology. What Young said to me and my fellow sociology undergraduates in the early 1980s was that, when it comes to crime, '*impossibilism*' had to be tackled. It is immoral to wait for major social change that might eradicate criminality while there were so many victims of crime now. I now make the case for *impossibilism* to be tackled in health.

Mental masturbation must give way to vigorous and applied intellectual intercourse, empirical evangelism must be assuaged by cultural sensitivity and epistemological suppleness, and asocial immoral localism must mature into socially moral globalism. *It is time to act!*

PRINCIPLES

Let me lay out some of the underlying realist[3] principles that I apply in this book:

1   Knowing what is real is problematic; but for some aspects of reality we have a 'workable' knowledge (such as cancer, AIDS, pain, and death); this workable realism is real enough for impotence to be replaced by action (for example, to alleviate human suffering).
2   'Consumers', 'customers', and 'users' are really 'patients' and we should stop wasting energy inventing politically correct euphemisms (most patients accept they are, and have no issue with being so described); 'health' services, policies, and problems are nothing of the sort, they are in reality 'disease' services, policies, and problems; patently, medical practitioners deal with disease, but so do most 'health' practitioners for most of their careers; collectively, medicine and the 'health' occupations, are therefore 'disciplines of disease'.[4]
3   Negative stereotyping of medical practitioners have them as arrogant and overpaid, and some in reality are incompetent, and one or two have been serial killers; but doctors are not really the enemy of the other disciplines of disease and sociologists, or patients, and the tendency to construe them as such (from whichever quarter) does little, if anything, to tackle the real enemy – disease and suffering.

4   Sociology isn't as silly as it seems: despite its reputation, jargon, the 'postmodern turn', and the dress-sense of many of its adherents, it can and should be not only a sceptical but an applied discipline with a paramount *raison d'être* to improve human reality.

5. Humans are living in, are influenced by, and interact with, a globalising society; global society is defined as the cultural, economic, and ecological interconnections, if not interdependence, of all human groupings); health/disease, therefore, is not just a local but a global social issue.

We know about and how to sort out the mess of the world. There is no excuse for inaction. As philosophical ethicist Peter Singer (2004) and revolutionary sociologist Slavoj Žižek (2008) declare, there are no innocent bystanders in a world of genocides, ecocides, famines, terrors, and diseases. Social scientists *and* the disciplines of disease have a moral obligation to address health/disease humanely and collegially through collective action.

FORMAT

This book, therefore, is about rehearsing what is known sociologically about health/disease and acting on that sociological knowledge.

Since the mid-1980s, I have taught sociology (applied to disease, madness, and murder) to doctors, nurses, midwives, health-visitors, social workers, physiotherapists, radiographers, occupational therapists, psychologists, pharmacists, and audiologists, as well as to students of sociology, social policy, criminology, education, law, chemistry, physics, and mathematics. It hasn't been easy.

As a consequence of this lengthy and testing teaching experience I have selected, from an extensive list of possibilities, subjects for the content of this book that are well cultivated within sociology, are topical, or which students have found most relevant. The starting point for a rigorous appreciation of any discipline must be its 'tools'. The chemist learns about periodic tables and how to make little bangs in the laboratory, the physicist about the laws of mass and motion as well as about a really big bang, the mathematician about geometrical and algebraic formulae as well as how to fill up a blackboard with numbers, and the physiologist about the anatomy and physiology of organs, molecules, and DNA, as well as how to cut up frogs. The sociologist has to learn about perspectives (theories, concepts, and research methodologies) that can be used as perceptual scalpels to slice open the guts of conventional wisdom.

Such learning is never easy. Ignorance is revealed, preconceptions disputed, and unfamiliar and difficult ideas are presented. The struggle and discomfort from thinking cannot be avoided. In the social sciences neither can the labour of reading widely. Moreover, while trying to limit jargon and aiming for clarity, I do not intend to 'dumb-down' difficult ideas or language (despite many of my students asking me to do so). There is already too much dumbing-down in academia, and plenty of dumb books which contain lots of made-simple diagrams and undemanding exercises to suitably patronise the pedestrian rather than provoke the keen. Furthermore, I have avoided over-referencing as it is both distracting for the reader and can be mere academic chauvinism rather than a necessary requirement for academic credibility. Statistics have also been kept to a minimum because in this informational age such data become quickly out-of-date (particularly in books) and is readily available via the Internet. Two accessible Internet sites for statistical data on topics covered in this book are that of the World Health Organization and the United Nations. As with all statistics, however, caveat emptor!

For those established sociologists (the subsidiary target reader-ship), much of the territory covered here will be familiar. However, the fashioning and packaging is not customary, and there are topics that are not usually covered in introductory 'sociology of health' books (for example, misery and murder). What is unique is the antagonistic tone towards my occupational superiors. I am match-lessly foolhardy in biting the providers of my intellectual succour. I am realistic to know that any mark I make will be no more than a gnat-bite on the *corps sociologique*. But sometimes the small bite of a gnat can make a bitten body move its position.

Suggestions for further reading have been included at the end of each chapter. Furthermore, each chapter also contains submissions for action – without action, thinking (and biting) are wasted. These are only my suggestions. What is important morally is to take action that benefits the health of one or more humans, and therefore, before taking any action, checks need to be made to ensure as far as possible that whatever you do is productive and not counter-productive. It need not be a grand gesture. Money given to charity agencies may be spent more on bureaucracy, conferences in five-star hotels, and brand-new four-wheel drive SUVs, than on actual human suffering. Taking a gap year or career break and travelling by jumbo jet to a distant village to build a toilet or teach English have more costs than benefits to both the planet and humanity. I implore you to do some research. For example (and this could be your first step towards moral action), listen to the BBC World Service (available on DAB and the Internet) and learn about what is happening in global society, and take part in the BBC's global conversations and debates. If you can, consult with your potential recipients. When I and my partner visited Zambia in 2003, what many of the children we met and their parents said they needed were pencils. Pencils gave the young the chance to get an education. I always carry pencils whenever I visit Africa, although I'm also open to other pencil-like insights into what can make a real difference to people's lives.

Chapter 1: Sociology   The *sociological imagination* is considered. This is the general approach used by sociologists to understand the world that is distinguishable from, for example, medical science or Buddhism. An overview is then provided of four key sociological perspectives: *structuralism*; *interactionism*; *constructionism/post-modernism*); and *realism*.

Chapter 2: Health   Competing definitions of health/disease are examined (as is the value of wholegrain bread and the signifi-cance of corsets). *Objective disease* (medical-scientific) is compared with *subjective illness* (individualistic meanings). These are then contrasted with the notion of *social sickness* (metaphors; filth; inequalities).

Chapter 3: Science   The cultural spread of science (*scientism*) is considerable, and science underpins medical knowledge and prac-tice (and increasingly that of the other disease disciplines). But how robust is science and therefore *medicine*? Moreover, how robust is the challenge for epistemological supremacy from medicine's *snake-oil* competitors?

Chapter 4: Power   Power in disease-care settings is the 'elephant in the room' – despite its conspicuousness, patients, practitioners, and policy-makers either ignore its existence or reframe its denotation. A durable way in which medicine (and nursing and pharmacy) acts as a powerful agency of *social control* is through the sick role. Moreover, *professional power* is exercise by medicine more than any of the other disease disciplines, on occasions with murderous consequences.

Chapter 5: Medicalisation   One of the most long-serving theories to have arisen from sociology is that of *medicalisation*. Even doctors have come to accept the disabling effect of over-using medical intervention in people's lives: *iatrogenesis*. However, medicalisation has metamorphosed into all-encompassing *healthism* and *psychohealthism*.

Chapter 6: Madness   The ranks of the mad in global society are swelling hugely. But what is madness and who are the *mad people*? Is *medical madness* a legitimate condition caused by personal (psychological and biological) deficits, or a deviance that medicine is required to socially control? Is *social madness*, not personal madness, the most significant 'disease' of global society?

Chapter 7: Misery   Misery has become medicalised, and happiness made into a profitable commodity. But the purveyance of happiness, based on studies of *nuns*, *rectums*, and *slums*, and veneration of such countries as *Bhutan* and *Iceland* as well as *cyberspace*, is impractical and therefore foolish. Moreover, the attempt to ameliorate misery through *money*, *medication* or *psychotherapy* is both misguided and immoral.

Chapter 8: Sex   Sex is part of being human. It is also part of disease care and disease prevention. Moreover, doctors and nurses have sexualised identities (probably unjustifiably). Patients have sexual needs (mostly unsatisfied). Biologists and sociology have a lot to say about sex (some of which is stupid). However, disease-care practitioners, patients, biologists, and sociologists could learn a lot from 'the wisdom of whores'.

Chapter 9: Death Everyone is going to die. *Social death* refers to how the social position and geographical location of the person concerned will affect how and when death occurs, and how both dying and death are perceived. However, because of globalisation, there is a tendency towards perceptual and administrative homogeneity regarding dying and death, and a relentless experience of *virtual death*.

Conclusion A summary of the book's substantive themes and messages is made. The suggested actions for tidying up the mess of global disease are collated. Rapprochement between the disciplines of disease and social scientists is sought. A new social contract for global health/disease is proffered.

NOTES

1 Socio-twaddle is the sociological equivalent of psycho-babble (the nonsensical obfuscation of commonsensical notions about human performance) in psychology and psychotherapy. Sociologists, including myself, have an obsessive compulsion to invent 'isms' and 'ists' – they/we are pre-eminent 'jargonists' spreading the linguistic malady of 'jargonism'.

2 The term 'human performance' is adapted from sociologist Erving Goffman (1959). Goffman was referring to the 'drama' of social life in which humans play their multiple parts. Here I am referring to all that makes humans human, their thoughts, actions, and emotions.

3 Confusion over the terms 'real', 'realist', 'realism', 'reality' is inevitable because these terms are used in everyday language as well as by sociologists; neither the laity nor academia can claim jurisdiction over these terms. I have tried to define here what I mean by 'realism', and further in Chapter 1, but undoubtedly will have failed to be consistent, thereby adding to the confusion.

4 This is so whether the practitioner operates in hospital or in the community. Midwifery and obstetrics may appear to focus on 'healthy' childbirth. However, as childbirth in the West has been medicalised, midwifery and obstetrics are 'disease' disciplines. Medical and nursing practitioners who provide inoculations and vaccinations also fall within the 'disease' bracket. Rather than health-enhancing, such practice is disease-preventing. These practitioners therefore abide by the philosophy and rules of disease.

SOCIOLOGY

1

IMAGINATION

. . . to understand the changes of many personal milieux we are required to look beyond them . . . To be able to do that is to possess the sociological imagination.

(Mills, 1959: 10–11)

AN ELDERLY WOMAN DIES ALONE from hypothermia in a run-down quarter of Atlanta, USA; a retired female architect celebrates the birth of her third great-grandson at an expensive restaurant in a fashionable district of Sydney; a young drug-dealing male is shot dead in a riot over rising food prices in down-town Port-au-Prince, Haiti; a child dies a slow death from diarrhoea in rural Sierra Leone, a country where more than one in four children die before the age of five years; a British soldier returning from serving in Afghanistan is diagnosed with post-traumatic stress disorder after a suicide attempt; an obese middle-aged businessman from Beijing, China, contracts type-2 diabetes; a teenage girl from Montpelier in France becomes dangerously emaciated after following advice about body-image from a pro-anorexia Internet site; a male media executive undergoes a full-health/disease assessment at a private clinic in Frankfurt, Germany, and is diagnosed as 'worried-but-well'.

All of these health, disease, life and death events are 'personal'. However, they are also 'social'. That is, health and disease are social phenomena with social meanings, causes, and solutions. Indeed, any aspect of human performance can only be understood fully when considered in the wider social context. This is not to deny the 'personal' aspects of health/disease events but to situate them within a myriad of cultural, political, and economic parameters. Whether it is an elderly woman dying from hypothermia within the richest country in the world, a child dying from diarrhoea in one of the poorest countries, or a worried well executive paying for health reassurance, how his/her society is organised, its values, beliefs, norms, and mores have had their effects. Realising this is to engage the sociological imagination.

For the sociologist, human performance is not 'natural' or 'God-given'. Falling in love, committing a crime, academic attainment, contracting syphilis are all influenced by social factors. The basis of the 'sociological imagination' is to look beyond the obvious, and to dispute both our own preconceived ideas and those of others. This is of particular importance when those with power in society hold prejudicial views about already vulnerable and dispossessed people or have hidden political agendas.

For example, the President of the USA received some very positive publicity in 2008 regarding his government's financial support of agencies in Africa helping to prevent HIV:

George Bush: a good man in Africa. As he starts a five-nation tour, the US president is an unlikely hero to the poor of a continent ravaged by AIDS.

They may not be George Bush's natural constituency but Rwanda's prostitutes have good things to say about him. So do poor South Africans abandoned by their quixotic government, and doctors across Africa who otherwise regard the American president as a walking crime against humanity.

As Bush arrives in Africa today at the start of a five-country tour he will be welcomed chiefly for an initiative which has gone largely unnoticed outside the continent but which has saved the lives of more than a million people with HIV.

The $15bn (£7.6bn) President's Emergency Plan for AIDS Relief (Pepfar) is in its fifth year and has been hailed as a 'revolution' that

16

is transforming healthcare in Africa and has been praised as the
most significant aid programme since the end of colonialism.

(Chris McGreal, *Guardian*, 2008a)

However, to dig a bit deeper into the story, a very different version
of this policy can be found. This is what the critical (about politicians
and their policies) Internet magazine *CounterPunch* reported:

Imperialism's Second Front: Bush's Foreign Sex Policy

According to Dr. Paul Zeitz, executive director of the Global AIDS
Alliance, a Washington-based AIDS advocacy group, PEPFAR "is
failing to stop the global spread of AIDS and failing to help lead
the world to stop this deadly disease."

This apparently-successful spending model is compromised in
three important ways. First, at least a third of the monies targeted
for prevention must be spent on abstinence-until-marriage pro-
grams. Second, three-fourths of the monies allocated for treatment
must be spent on the purchase and distribution of antiretroviral
drugs from U.S. pharmaceutical manufactures and cannot be
substituted by generic alternatives. Finally, at least half of that
allocated for helping children and orphans is to be provided through
nonprofit, nongovernmental organizations, particularly faith-based
groups.

(David Rosen, *CounterPunch*, 2006)

The task for sociologists is to uncover (through theorising and
research) which version is more candid.

Moreover, the task of sociology must also be about attempting
to make society a better place for people, more humane, just, and
equitable. Therefore, simply being sceptical about Bush's policy is
unsatisfactory (morally). My definition of sociology is therefore:

Thinking about, questioning, *and* contributing to society.

The inauguration of sociology, an academic discipline, is attributed
to August Comte (1798–1857). However, most civilisations have
produced thinkers who questioned and wanted to improve society.
For example, Socrates, Plato, and Aristotle were all sociologically
minded (as well as philosophical and scientific).

17

C. Wright Mills (1959) galvanised academic sociology further with his recognition that 'private troubles' were also 'public issues'. The private trouble of the death of a loved one in a car accident is a public issue. Globally, each year 1.5 million people die on the roads. Every three minutes a child is killed on the roads. Most of those who die live/die in developing countries (Make Roads Safe, 2008). Such carnage (which is nothing short of genocide) is dependent upon: the amount of money governments put into road safety; how much the United Nations pressurises governments to implement road safety measures; the speed to which countries with emerging capitalist economies are modernising their infrastructures; and how much value a society places on private transport and on having commodities in retail outlets available on demand. Hence, politicians, the media, and you and I collude in this human road-killing because we are either apathetic about intervention or energetic about protecting our lifestyles.

The private trouble of having a cancerous tumour is also a public issue. How a society is organised economically and culturally will contribute to the contracting of the disease. For example, rapidly industrialising countries and those underdeveloped countries that service global corporations may not have appropriate health and safety regulations to protect workers from carcinogenic materials, nor for the disposal of those materials (World Health Organization, 2007). Moreover, in these countries the sale of cigarettes is not controlled by governments, and they are sold vigorously by tobacco companies (Sebrié and Glantz, 2006). In developed countries, funding for research into and the treatment of cancer may not be as high a budgetary or social priority as leisure, housing, or invading other countries, and certain cancers (for example, prostate and testicular) may be neglected while others are attended (for example, breast and cervical) because of traditional differences in gender-role performance. As with death on the roads, there is a general complicity in deaths from cancer because of interventional apathy or redirected energy.

As the work of Comte and Mills implies, along with the definition of the subject I have offered, social events and social relationships are not taken at face value by the sociologist. Conventional wisdom ('common sense') is tested to see whether or not it stands up to the scrutiny of systematic theorising and/or rigorous research. This is the role of any academic subject. For example, medical science disputed a previously prevailing lay belief in Western countries that 'stress' caused stomach ulcers, and disputes the present lay belief in parts of Africa that HIV/AIDS can be cured by having sex with a virgin.

However, the task that sociologists set themselves is to query all knowledge, including that of medical science, even when that knowledge is a criticism of other knowledge. For example, medicine was found to have overstated its claimed efficacy in reducing the incidence of death from infectious diseases in Europe during the nineteenth and twentieth centuries by epidemiologist Thomas McKeown (1976). McKeown identified in particular better sanitation and nutrition as crucial in lowering death rates rather than medical intervention (given that medical practitioners had significant involvement in improving sanitation and nutrition). But, as (sociologist) Sarah Nettleton (2006) records, his work in turn has been accused by a number of other sociologists of not accounting adequately for such social factors as improvements in workers' wages and the consequential alterations in the relations between social classes.

Theories are the key tools for sociological investigation, and four 'frameworks' are outlined here and applied in various guises throughout the book. These theoretical frameworks are collections of theories that may have subtle differences between them, but that have similar philosophical routes, and complementary observations to make about how society operates.

The first theoretical framework, *structuralism*, regards society having a set of configurations and an overall impact that induces humans to perform in preordained ways, including being healthy or diseased. At its extreme, structuralism considers human performance as completely 'determined' by society. The structural sociology accepts the existence of social facts (such as poverty and disease) and (empirical) science. Quantitative techniques such as the social survey are used to discover facts about society and support or undermine theory.

In opposition to structuralism, *interactionism*, the second explanatory framework, argues that humans have personal volition. For the interactionist, people interpret and give meaning to their lives. Hence, rather than being determined by society, people determine society. Although the interactionist does not accept that there are 'social facts', science is, as with structuralism, utilised. To ascertain the meanings and interpretations individuals and groups give to their lives, qualitative techniques such as participant observation and in-depth interviewing are employed and generate theory.

The *constructionist* position, which is the third theoretical framework, takes the interactionist stance much further by positing that reality is fabricated. At its (postmodernist) extreme, all of human performance, all social entities, all physical matter, and all scientific laws are considered merely socially accepted 'constructs'. This includes cancer, cholesterol, and cardiopathy. Consequently, constructionism either uses only theory or adopts and adapts, somewhat hypocritically, qualitative scientific method, given that science itself is considered a construct.

Lastly, *realism* combines the structuralist stance that there are social facts and natural facts, with the interactionist/constructionist view that interpretation and meaning have to be accommodated. For the realist, there are facts but they are hidden by a cloak of cultural denotations and symbols. Any scientific technique, or combined qualitative and quantitative methods, can be used by the realist. But the realist recognises that science and all other epistemologies have so far been inadequate in finding and explaining reality.

STRUCTURALISM

The structural paradigm in sociology posits that humans belong to social groups and that it is membership of these groups that to a greater or lesser degree dictates human performance. For the structuralist, social institutions, society, and social divisions set out the constraints and boundaries for human performance. These social institutions include the organisations and systems of disease care, criminal justice, educational, commerce, leisure, travel, media, as well as the family. Society is divided by social class, gender, ethnicity, age, and geographical region, as well by levels of poverty/wealth, power/subjugation, and health/disease.

Structuralist theorising has infiltrated many areas of local and global disease-care policy. There is an acceptance both in principle and policy by governments, the World Health Organization, the United Nations, and the World Bank that reductions in disease rely solely or heavily on structural change. This applies to particular cultures and to global society.

For Comte (1798–1857), there were general laws of social structure and development just as the chemist or physicist was able to state that laws existed in the physical world and thereby shaped that world. He perceived society as analogous to human anatomy and physiology. All structures of society like the structures of the human body (for example, the heart, liver, brain, and colon) were interconnected. Each was dependent on the other parts, and this was to become more so as society progressed through its historical stages towards greater complexity. By the twenty-first century the body is of gigantean proportions – the colossus of global society.

Preordained patterns of society are maintained by various ideologies: economic, political, cultural, and religious systems of belief. Capitalism, communism, and Christianity are examples of doctrines that recommend, if not dictate, how people should think, behave, and feel. Ideological messages (blatant, subliminal, seductive, and bullying) about self-responsibility, self-betterment, the body-beautiful and the blissful mind, are compiled by the powerful and endorsed by the agencies of the state and the media. These messages present a 'normative' set out of values, which the 'good citizen' is expected (and may be forced) to follow. What is being communicated through a mixture of explicit and implicit, verbal, non-verbal, printed and electronic transmissions are the rules for acceptable performance. Those who don't abide by the rules, if they are found out, become denounced as 'deviants' or 'antisocial', thereby attracting the social control mechanisms of approbation and punishment. Deviancy includes disease, and therefore disease is susceptible to social control.

Comte's sociological 'holism' proposes that not only is society made up of interrelated parts, but it is greater than the sum of its parts. Every human is made up of billions of molecules, genes, and DNA, but it is not possible to understand humanity or even an individual human by examining the constituent elements of an individual. Microscopic examination of tissues along with genetic mapping, of course, reveals much about how humans operate. However, this is not enough to comprehend the personality, physique, and temperament of an individual, let alone why there are differences between humans. The effect of a full orchestra playing and choir, replete with sopranos, altos, tenors, and basses, singing *The Messiah* in the Carnegie Hall, Sydney Opera House, or Royal Albert Hall, is not discernible from scanning Handel's notation. Similarly, for Comte, an understanding of society cannot be achieved by focusing on the performance of humans as individuals, or by aggregating these performances.

Emile Durkheim (1858–1917), greatly influenced by Comte, developed the theme of holism into a strain of structuralism called *functionalism*. Functionalism regards all social institutions as having a purpose, and in the main this purpose is beneficial to society. As society changes, so do the social institutions in order maintain their beneficial functions.

For example, the social institution of the family has the function of socialising children into the norms of society. But if these norms alter (and they have done so in many parts of the world), so does the composition of the family. For example, the composition of the family varies greatly across the world due in large part to the shift towards a global capitalist economy, but also because of diseases such as HIV/AIDS and more liberal attitudes towards sexuality (nuclear, step, lone-parent, and gay/lesbian families increasing at the expense of extended family arrangement whether patriarchal or matriarchal). The social institutions of law enforcement (the police and courts) have the function of sustaining social stability. As new threats to that stability surface (for example, terrorism, sex-tourism, and cybercrime), or old ones are given greater attention (for example, race-hate, neighbourhood noise, and school truancy), then police officers and the judiciary readjust how they operate to contain the threat. The social institution of the university formerly had the function of generating knowledge for its own sake along with (allegedly) cultural and competent leaders for the arts and politics. But universities, except for a few high-ranking institutions, have turned into 'knowledge assembly lines' to facilitate an ever more complex division of labour for the global capitalist economy (including the 'service industries' of medicine, nursing, and the other disciplines of disease).

For Durkheim, sociological research should seek out social facts, and use methods (specifically, the social survey) that can illuminate the structural impositions of society on human performance. Durkheim, like all structuralists, rejects the 'reductionist' view that social acts (for example, getting married, being ill, and working as a doctor or nurse) can be explained by reference to individual motivation.

A major contribution made by Durkheim to the stucturalist argument is his empirical study of suicide (Durkheim, 1966; orig. 1897). Comparing cross-societal rates of suicide, Durkheim argued that the structure of society is crucial to decisions about taking one's life. While he accepts that for some people there was individual choice, a state of 'normlessness' (Durkheim's term was 'anomie'), engendered by an absence of systems of social support and strong belief systems, increased the likelihood of suicide. In those countries where family and religion were important, people had tangible norms to give their lives poignancy, shape, and direction.

Durkheim's proposition about the social nature of suicide has been criticised for taking official figures as reliable. Data in countries where the family and religion are more respected as social institutions may be massaged to hide the actual level of suicide (Pope, 1976).

Functionalism can also be criticised for not recording the negative effects of social institutions on society. For example: the abuse that occurs in families; the police and the courts serving the interests of the ruling elite; universities used to 'mop up' the unemployed; and the disciplines of disease distracting attention from a core cause of morbidity and mortality – society.

A further criticism of functionalism is that it only offers a circular ('teleological') description rather than a deep analysis. For example, answering the question 'why are most nurses women?', a functionalist might reply that 'women are most suited to nursing work'. If then asked the question 'what work most suits women?', the answer might be 'nursing'. There is, therefore, little appreciation of other issues that need to be considered such as (from a feminist perspective) the way in which the historical subjugation of women has pushed them into relatively menial and subordinate work compared with men.

Notwithstanding inherent deficiencies in functionalist reasoning, Comte and Durkheim's view that social structure affects human performance dramatically is a momentous one. However, Karl Marx (1818–1883), along with his co-theorist, Friedrich Engels (1820–1895), offers a different version of structuralism from that

23

of functionalists (although there are functionalist elements to most structuralist perspectives). Marx's 'conflict' or 'critical' structuralism emphasises the fundamental importance of the economy in shaping human performance.

Marx's investigation of the intricacies, corruptions, and conflicts in capitalism remain highly relevant to twenty-first century globalised society. Moreover, his understanding of the detrimental effects of capitalism on human health is still pertinent.

In his early publications Marx (1959; orig. 1844) argued that the way capitalist society was structured caused people to become 'alienated' from their own humanity. Work, for Marx, was core to being human. Work allowed individuals to express their creativity, and encouraged cooperation between humans and within society. This observation has functionalist overtones.

However, Marx argued that the consequence of the capitalist way of working was to undermine creativity, and substitute social cooperation with interpersonal rivalry and exploitation. Within the capitalist mode of production (his term for an economic system) humans are no longer in control of their work and therefore their humanity is debased. Economies based on local agriculture and small-scale businesses maintain the connection between humans and work. Industrialisation, urbanisation, and the move to employment in large-scale industrial factories result in 'employees' becoming estranged from what they produce and a loss of job satisfaction. Work is no longer rewarding but a time-controlled toil for others in return for money. In Marxist terms, workers have become 'wage slaves'.

The epitome of alienated work in industrial settings was the twentieth-century car 'assembly line'. A worker would have one small task to perform repeatedly without any need to comprehend how this fitted into the overall car design. By the twenty-first century, much of this repetitive and insentient labour was being conducted by robots. However, computers were also responsible for the growth in another form of alienated work. There has been a huge growth in the number of computer operatives who sit in large 'office-warehouses' dealing with insurance, banking, travel, and telecommunications. For example, globally, tens of millions of people are employed in call centres. The modern sweat-shop, like its forerunner, is characterised by low wages, debt-bondage, over-crowded and unsafe conditions. Furthermore, industrialising countries with rapidly emerging economies (principally China and India) are recreating the miserable, insecure, degrading, and abusive conditions that Engels described in 1845 about the English working class (Engels, 1999; orig. 1892).

Marx in his later work, the seminal text *Das Kapital* (1971; orig. 1867), highlighted the connection between the economic 'base' of a society and what makes up the rest of society (its 'superstructure'). The economic base is made up of: (a) the particular mode of production (examples of which are: ancient; feudal; agrarian; capitalist); (b) the machinery and technology used in the production of goods and services (the 'means of production'); (c) and two groupings of people. These groupings consist of, on the one hand, the people who do the work, and on the other, those who force them to do so, or employ them. According to Marx, throughout history these two groups have been in tension with one another. In ancient society it was slaves against the free citizens, in medieval times it was feudal nobility against the serfs, and in the industrial age the proletariat (the working class) against the bourgeoisie (the middle class).

The superstructure of a society is all the other institutions (for example: religion; the family; disease-care systems; education; criminal justice; politics; media; and therapy) and their concomitant belief and practices. That is, what people feel, do, and think is inspired by the economic system.

Marx argued that it was the conflict between the 'exploited' and the 'exploiters' in each type of economic system that led to change. He anticipated that capitalism would eventually change, either through evolution or revolution (depending on which interpretation of Marx's writing is adopted), into an economic system without exploitation (that is, to a communist mode of production).

Exploitation occurs for Marx under capitalism through forcing people to work in dangerous and filthy surroundings with monotonous jobs, and with no power to influence the running of the factory or business. However, his significant contribution to the study of economics was to identify how the bourgeoisie exploited the proletariat. He realised that an employee may produce goods worth a certain amount when these goods are sold, but received much less than that amount as wages. The rest, the 'surplus value', was the profit for the bourgeoisie.

Crucially, for Marx, the economic base directs the shape and denotation of everything else in society (that is, the superstructure). For Marx, the capitalist form of economy is supported by an ideology that favours the interests of the bourgeoisie (which for Marx in nineteenth-century Europe, was also the ruling class).

However, Marx's prediction that social progress would be obtained through the ascendancy of socialism and then communism appears discredited. The 'Communist Block' of Eastern Europe and the Soviet Union collapsed in 1991. By 2008, only the Republic of Cuba and the Democratic People's Republic of (North) Korea retained their Marxist economic credentials. China and Vietnam have developed novel forms of capitalism in which politically they are socialist/communist but are economically capitalist. Moreover, China has the prospect of global (capitalist) economic dominance by the middle of the twenty-first century. The exceptions are Venezuela where Hugo Chavez, elected president in 1999, has been attempting to readjust his country's capitalist system towards socialism, and in Nepal where in April 2008 the Maoist Communist Party appeared to have won a majority of seats in the elections to the constitutional assembly. However, Marx's attachment to any of the adaptations of his ideas cannot be assured. It is possible, if not probable, that he would stand by the statement 'if that's communism then I'm not a communist' attributed apocryphally to him.

Marx envisaged that capitalism, like all other economic systems, would eventually collapse due to its 'internal contradictions'. The swings in employment and unemployment, the ultimate limit to available markets, the spreading of wars to defend existing markets, and the increase in trade union activity collectivising the demands of working peoples would be the catalysts.

However, far from being defeated, today capitalism is pandemic, cutting across national boundaries. The globalisation of capitalism, according to Marxist Antonio Gramsci (1971), is maintained through the dissemination of a virulent and highly politicised ideology – 'hegemony'. Western-based (largely USA) economic philosophies have spread commodity fetishism and the mystification of reality to nearly every country. Western values concerning, for example, material possession, employment, and health/disease to societies with other cultural practices are becoming normalised in global society. Moreover, mass electronic communication systems and media, along with international tourism, serve to increase the rate and depth of the Western practices into other cultures. 'Corporate capitalism', whereby economic control is in the hands of the executives and major shareholders of complex transnational businesses and financial institutions, is taking over from local and national capitalist enterprise.

There has not only been a globalisation of Western culture, but also of Western inequalities (Glyn, 2006). Wealth is not shared equally between the developed (Western), developing (transitional/emerging), and underdeveloped (stagnating/declining) countries of the world, or within these countries. The widening intersocietal and intrasocietal inequality gap has produced a global elite, extracting surplus value from a globalised workforce. Both the elite and the workforce are increasingly itinerant, the former moving to areas of the world where trade can be conducted with minimal restrictions and costs, and the latter searching for employment wherever it can be found. In a hegemonised global society, the Chinese and Indian bourgeoisie culturally have more in common with their counterparts in Europe, Australasia, and North America than they do with their fellow non-elite citizens.

However, the most pertinent 'social facts' to underline the persistent relevance of Marx in the twenty-first century are: about 40 per cent of the world's population lives on less than US$2 per day (United Nations, 2008); the combined wealth of Warren Buffett, Carlos Slim Helu, Bill Gates, and Lakshm Mittal, the world's four wealthiest people, is US$223 billion (Forbes, 2008); and the financial system that underwrites global capitalism has come close to collapse (*Financial Times*, 2008).

INTERACTIONISM

Max Weber (1864–1920) challenged structuralism, particularly Marxism, with his interactionist sociological perspective. As with structuralism, many other sociological theories owe their origins to his work (for example, constructionism/postmodernism).

For Weber (1948), humans have consciousness and free will, and this allows them to interpret their experiences. Metals, planets,

27

protons, cars, neutrons, grass, and air do not think and reflect. This makes the study of human society a very different task from that of studying the natural world and human-made objects – that is, until 'bio-computers' produce a fully operational combination of the inanimate and animate.

Humans have choices, argues Weber, and they elect constantly (although not necessarily consistently) to act on those choices. However, this is not a replication of psychological reductionism. For Weber, humans are not made up of an individual psychology operating in a social vacuum. Weber regards humans as inexorably connected to the social setting in which they live out their daily lives, as well as to the broader society to which they belong. They give meaning to their lives. The meaning they give to their lives, however, is married to their social situation and is not divorced from it, as much of psychology implies (notable exceptions being Freudian and social learning theories).

Weber suggests that the meaning individuals give to their action is what creates society (this he termed 'social actionism'). Society is not, as Durkheim would have it, 'greater than the sum of its parts', but is only 'the sum of its parts'. That is, people react to their environment, and offer interpretations of social events. Therefore, people consciously make and alter the social order around them, rather than, as the structuralists propose, having society impinging on human free will.

Weber rejected 'objective' sociological methods of research. He argued for an 'interpretative' method through which the sociologist would intuitively or empathetically come to understand human behaviour and therefore the working of society. The German word *verstehen* is commonly utilised to describe this thorough comprehension of the meaning that social actors give to their behaviour. Participant observation is the Weberian research method of choice (although in-depth interviewing is frequently used as a more practical alternative). Here the researcher deliberately enters the world of the people he/she wishes to study. Weber argued that it is only possible to appreciate fully (or as fully as possible) what is happening in any given social situation if you become part of it. At both the individual level, at the larger group level, and the structural level, individual and collective interpretations of situations must be understood – then the sociologist has achieved *verstehen*.

Weber disagrees with Marx over the power of the economy base to dictate human performance. He points to elements of the super-structure of society (specifically, religious belief) operating as the catalyst for change rather than the economic base. Against Marx's 'historical materialism' (that is, history changes on the basis of whatever economic system is forming), Weber argued that it was the 16th-century Protestant Reformation in Europe that stimulated the growth of the capitalist mode of production. Specifically, it was the beliefs of the Protestant Calvinists that brought about capitalism.

Calvinists valued hard work and individual achievement. They thought that if their work endeavours were successful and as individuals they advanced in society, then this indicated that God had selected them to enter heaven on death. Crucially, the wealth they accrued could not be spent on 'conspicuous consumption' (which would be sinful), but should be reinvested in business and commerce. This had the effect, reasoned Weber, of building up the industrial economies of Europe, which then stimulated capitalist growth in other parts of the world.

Weber also disagreed with Marx over who had power in society. For Marx, the locus of power is found in whichever class controlled the means of production, whether the mode of production was ancient, agrarian, feudal, or capitalist. However, Weber believed that people other than those with economic supremacy could hold power in society. Weber's point is that certain 'status groups' may have more esteem and influence than, for example, the wealthy people. In liberal democracies, an individual born into the bottom of the social hierarchy can (in theory) rise to the top by gaining educational and professional qualifications. The daughter of a shopkeeper would become Prime Minister of Britain, and the son of a peanut farmer President of the United States of America. Winning the lottery might not mean automatic entry into the power-elite of a society, but will alter the social prestige of the winner or his/her offspring.

In particular, Weber and Weberian theorists such as Elliot Freidson (1970; 1971) argue that collections of people have the potential to employ strategies in order to increase their control over their own work, gain greater remuneration, and thereby socially advance. The medical and legal professions have done this successfully. Nursing, physiotherapy, occupational therapy, audiology, and clinical psychology are attempting to repeat this process with differential degrees of success. The technique used by such groups, argued Weber, is that of 'social closure'. In order to advance the status of a group its leaders make it increasingly difficult to belong to that group by elevating the requirements for entry. Furthermore, the claim is advanced by the group that only *its* members have the authority and expertise to operate in a well-defined area of work (such as surgery and prescribing, and legal representation and judgement).

Weber's sociology has made notable contributions to social policy. For example, most disease-prevention programmes in Western countries and those advocated by the World Health Organization (WHO) now modify the crude 'finger-wagging' approach of telling people how to live less diseased lives (for example, stop smoking, stop binge-drinking, stop eating fatty, sugary, and salty foods, and stop being lazy). It has become an acceptable part of health-promotion policies to try to understand why certain social groups persist in unhealthy actions, and to try to accommodate the meanings people attach to their actions (while still steering them towards changing them, of course).

Interactionist Erving Goffman (1959) has contributed to both sociology and to how certain people and groups in society are (badly) regarded. Goffman, using his 'dramaturgy' perspective, considers human 'performance' as a drama. He argues that society produced guidelines (social scripts) for how people should act in their many roles. These scripts are shaped by the social and physical environment. In particular, scripts are affected by the 'symbolic' reactions of the audience and the reaction people had to the audience. The environment and the audience provide blatant parameters for what Goffman calls the 'front-stage' performance (for example, written codes of behaviour, consistent positive or negative feedback), while also transmitting rules for the performance obliquely. The front-stage scene is what is presented in public. However, there are also elements to the role being played that are hidden from public view in the 'back-stage' scene. These elements are the rehearsals, secrets, and deviances of the role.

For example, nurses, when faced with the prospect of front-stage confrontation with doctors, may enact the back-stage 'doctor–nurse game' involving passive–aggressive non-cooperation (Stein, 1967;

Reeves *et al.*, 2008). An associated tactic used to deal with front-stage pressures from colleagues, as well as demands from patients and hospital bureaucracy, is to engage in their 'subculture of complaints' backstage, which involves bonding with peers through whingeing about their mutual plight (Turner, 1986).

The emergence of globalised mass electronic communication has opened the drama of human performance to the virtual world. Electronic mail, online chat rooms, and specialist Internet services (such as those delivering medical advice) all without face-to-face interaction, carry novel forms of symbolic feedback. In electronic communication the boundaries between front-stage and backstage areas of a performance become blurred.

The practitioner–patient session is a drama. Consider the front-stage: the clinic or hospital entrance conveys selective information to the patient: its decor, its serene or manic tone. The prestige and power of the doctor is garnered through the symbols of medical professionalism. Backstage, however, the interminable tribalism of the disease disciplines will be playing, and other, perhaps less respectful, discussions about the patient.

Goffman also described how some people undergo 'spoiled identities' because of the stigma they attract from physical, psychological, or social labels that carry negative connotations. An individual may be perceived and respond as not 'normal' or 'whole'. If the individual receives feedback consistently from others that he/she is somehow 'damaged', then self-worth becomes undermined. A diagnosis of schizophrenia, depression, epilepsy, and HIV/AIDS, having a speech defect, facial disfigurement, or a disabled limb, and being convicted of paedophilia or rape, may all attract stigma and thereby spoiled identities.

CONSTRUCTIONISM

The interactionist notion that individuals give meaning to their lives is readjusted by constructionist theorists. For the constructionist, the social world does not exist as such. The meanings humans make of their lives and of aspects of society feel 'real' only because humans have decided that they should be real. For Peter Berger and Thomas Luckmann (1967) reality is socially constructed.

The constructionist view of health and disease, therefore, is that it is socially manufactured. Any state of health or disease does not exist without humans deciding to make them exist and providing descriptions of them. Whereas the medical scientist believes that diseases are real and can be identified and described as 'facts', the constructionist argues that they only have the appearance of having a reality because of the coming together of certain historical and social processes. At other times, and in other places, they would either not be construed as real at all or they would be interpreted as different entities.

There is a link between 'cultural relativism' and constructionism. Social phenomena, for the constructionist, are understood on the basis of the values of a particular culture. Consequently, cultural practices in one society cannot have any essential 'rightness' or 'wrongness', nor can they be 'better' or 'worse' than those of another culture. Each culture can only be assessed on its own terms. Hence, the ritualistic expunging of the clitoris in young North African women, the pervasive use of the death penalty in China, human rights abuses in Middle-Eastern countries, or the binge-drinking and sexual liberalism of British and Australian youth can only be judged from within those cultures and not externally. Cultural relativism disallows universals in normality and morality.

An offshoot of constructionism is 'labelling theory' based on the notion that labels affect profoundly social attitudes and self-identity. It is, therefore, closely related to the (symbolic) interactionism of Erving Goffman. Moreover, as with Goffman's work, labelling theory has application to health/disease.

Labelling theory examines what becomes categorised as 'deviance' in society, including criminality, madness, and some physical conditions. Theorists who employ the labelling approach consider what society describes as deviance not as inherent to the biological or psychological make-up of the individual. Rather, some sets of actions or beliefs attract the tag of 'deviancy' (Lemert, 1951; Becker, 1963). What the labelling theorists argue is that no element of human performance is ever either 'normal' or 'abnormal' until that meaning has been ascribed to it by others, especially powerful others. Car theft, burglary, or even rape and murder are not crimes until the criminal justice system declares them to be so. Eating too much, drinking too much, smoking, and being indolent are not abhorrent behaviours until the 'health police' (which, of course, is another value-laden label) decide they are.

A distinction is made between primary and secondary stages of labelling. Rule-breaking has only a negligible effect on how rule-breakers perceive themselves or are viewed by others. This is especially the case if our deviancy is unnoticed by the powerful, but if our actions are uncovered and the reaction of others is marked, we might begin a 'deviant career' (Goffman, 1963). The secondary stage of labelling is entered whereby, because of consistent reinforcement of the label, a permanent deviant identity is forged. The label then starts to define the person, and he/she internalises the performance that is connected to that label. Furthermore, the process of becoming a complete deviant is enhanced if the individual socialises with groups who have been given similar labels. In particular, what Goffman (1961) describes as 'total institutions', such as gaols and asylums, will reinforce a criminal or mad identity.

A patient (which is also a label that carries particular expectations, some of which are negative) diagnosed with diabetes or having suffered a cerebro-vascular accident will soon after diagnosis begin to internalise the characteristics of that label. No matter that he/she does not immediately perform as a diabetic or stroke victim, there will be little escape from the socialisation process initiated by the general practitioner or medical consultant and reinforced by nurses, physiotherapists, the individual's family, friends, and work colleagues, and perhaps too much information downloaded from the Internet. Eventually, he/she will enter to the second stage of labelling and become a 'diabetic' or 'stroke victim'.

So, the tenet of constructionism is that reality is not reality but only what society (or certain sections of society) decides is reality. But this does not mean that these made-up realities are not experienced as real. Humans construct their realities by objectifying subjective experience (Berger and Luckman,1967). Social phenomena are imbibed with culturally pertinent value and utility. They therefore have a (constructed) vital capacity which is both produced by society and is necessary for society to operate. We live our lives as though health, disease, death, war, money, happiness, misery have tangible existence.

However, some extremist constructionists (the postmodernist sociologists) have made it their business not only to deconstruct each and every one of these realities, but to leave them in a state of disintegration. Reality thus destroyed is left to fester or be recreated in a multiplicity of styles.

For the postmodernist, everything in both the social world *and* the physical world is merely a product of the human mind. There are no, and can never be any, universal laws or incontrovertible established facts. Truth of any sort, therefore, is not possible – ever. The 'grand narratives' of nationhood, Christianity, Islam, Judaism, socialism, capitalism, and science that purported to explain the social, physical, or spiritual world are all only systems of belief (as is postmodernism). Furthermore, the demise in deference towards politicians, teachers, the police, the judiciary, the clergy, and academics is indicative of this postmodern 'reality'.

Consequently, there is no good, bad, right, or wrong way for humans to live their lives. There is in the postmodern world a cultural marketplace that has reconstructed humans as consumers and all things as commodities (including health, happiness, holidays, sex, entertainment, leisure, and death).

In the postmodern health/disease-market, the herbalist, homeopath, aromatherapist, astrologist, and gynaecologist, have equal legitimacy, ranging from none to absolute, depending on the disposition of the consumer.

An open choice about lifestyle, and what we want to do, feel, and think, can be considered the ultimate in personal empowerment. Michel Foucault, pre-empting postmodernist theorising, argued that absolute freedom for an individual could only be obtained by revealing and removing all social constraints on thought, knowledge, and behaviour. Through his 'archaeological' social scientific investigative technique, he revealed that all knowledge (and hence thinking) was inhibited by the interests of the powerful in society. He concluded that all knowledge was relative, thereby removing the control the powerful had over others (Foucault, 1969). To reveal and remove social limitations on behaviour he took hard drugs, and also indulged in uninhibited acts such as 'suicidal orgies'. These disputations with death involved risky homosexual and sadomasochist practices in Californian 'parlours' (West, 2004). For Foucault, the ultimate control over one's life was gained by not fearing death. James Miller, in his review of Foucault's life and work, records Foucault's response to an undergraduate student's question about personal autonomy while he was lecturing at the University of California in 1983:

> Who could be scared of AIDS? You could be hit by a car tomorrow. Even crossing the street was dangerous! If sex with a boy gives me pleasure – why renounce such pleasure? We have the power . . . we shouldn't give it up.
>
> (Foucault, quoted in Miller, 1993: 353)

Alternatively, such liberation, if it doesn't result in death (Foucault died a year later from an AIDS-related disease), may induce catastrophic anxiety over what and who we are. Vulnerability to socially provoked 'ontological insecurity', whereby we become chronically unsure of our 'self', is pandemic. However, whereas in the West and among the bourgeoisie of emerging countries angst about the meaning of one's own existence has replaced insecurities concerning survival, in underdeveloped countries it is superimposed on survival concerns. That is, people living in impoverishment have to worry about obtaining clean water and the rising price of basic foodstuffs as well as being subjected to the seductions of a materialist lifestyle. The rural and urban poor may struggle to obtain the basic necessities of life, but nevertheless they are likely to have access to televisions and pass huge billboards along the highways and in towns that promote luxury cars, exotic holidays, and high-fashion as 'normal'.

REALISM

Sociology comprises a family of theories, conjugated by the understanding that the society and human performance are linked. However, this family is split with structuralism in one camp and constructionism in the other, as well as interactionism (postmodernism being the demon child who has escaped from the epistemological attic and imposed itself on the latter). Realism acts as a family therapist in this internecine feud.

Realism in social science is a misleading term as it does not mean what it implies in everyday usage. For the realist, social scientist (and there are, as with the other frameworks, different kinds of social scientific realism) 'real' entities do exist in the natural and social world that may eventually become known and understood. That is, realism accepts that in the natural world there are concrete objects and universal laws, but as yet establishing what the reality of these entities is has not yet been achieved through science (or any other epistemology).

The failure to understand reality is first caused by the 'culture overlay' on reality. Second, social and natural scientific techniques to date are inadequate for the task of uncovering reality, although we do get glimpses at reality occasionally. Science can offer a 'best guess' of what these objects are and how the world operates. Third, the realist also acknowledges that humans can only experience these subjectively and therefore can never 'know' anything in its purest form. Establishing truth in the social and natural world, therefore, is severely hindered by society, science, and our 'selves'.

Crucial to the realist position on social reality is reflexivity. Humans, argue realists, have a reflexive relationship with society. That is, humans are shaped by their social world (the structuralist position), and help shape their social world (the constructionist/ interactionist position). What individuals feel, do, and think affects the content and form of their societies. An individual's emotions, behaviours, and cognition are affected by the content and form of his/her society.

Consequently, neither the human performance nor society remains static. Changes in both, while not necessarily random and amorphous (individuals and society both have restrictions on their malleability: biology and language restrict humans, and social structures restrict society), are not unitary or linear but complex and multidirectional. Therefore, profound alterations in human performance and in society are difficult, if not impossible, to predict despite the exuberant claims of behavioural and cognitive psycho-therapists and social-engineering politicians. However, in the future, sociology, political science, medical science, and psychology, or other disciplines yet not conceived might be able to be compre-hend fully and prophesise accurately human performance and the functioning of society.

The continuous rearranging and updating of social and scientific knowledge, periodic epistemological paradigm shifts, and contradictory findings from research studies are indicative of the relatively primitive methods available for discovering reality. 'Research suggests', a stock phrase of the empiricist, is followed by another stock phrase, 'however, further research is needed'. It is likely that the further research contradicts the original research, so the public is left mystified and cynical: is alcohol good or bad for health? If so, how much and what type is good or bad? What is the normal level of cholesterol and blood pressure, and bodyweight ration? How much exercise should be taken – twenty minutes a day or an hour a day? However, amid the confusion over accurate knowledge some facts do surface: smoking kills; starvation kills; malaria kills; HIV/AIDS kills; guns kill; vaccinations protect against polio and smallpox; people in developed countries on average live much longer than people in underdeveloped countries.

Realist Roy Bhaskar (2008) has talked of the discrepancy between what we think we know about society and nature (what social and natural scientists claim as evidence of reality) and actual knowledge. For Bhaskar there are two forms of knowledge. First, there is what he describes as 'intransitive knowledge', which is made up of the invariable and inviolable facts that exist with or without our knowledge of them. Second, there is transitive knowledge, which is made up of the language, concepts, and technologies of the epistemological discourse that is afforded the credibility in a specific culture or epoch to tackle reality. Today, it is science that dominates as an explanatory paradigm, but because it is obvious that science does not understand many areas of social and natural life (that is, science has only retrieved minimal intransitive knowledge), a conglomeration of major and minor religions and 'alternative' therapies compete with science.

However, does it matter that intransitive knowledge remains obscure? That is, should society be worried about not having access to 'truth'?

Sociologist Frank Furedi (2004) argues that the social role of the intelligentsia should be the search for truth. However, intellectual pursuit of the truth has been undermined if not lost because universities have become too bureaucratic, overmanaged, orientated to work rather than ideas (Morrall, 2009). Ophelia Benson and Jeremy

Stangroom (2006) attack what they describe as the 'assorted political and ideological agendas' in academia (and in particular those with a postmodernism bent) that have made truth unfashionable. For them, distrust and disdain for truth is based on a deliberate misinterpretation of science:

> It is arguable that obfuscation is what postmodernism is all about. Clouds of squid ink in the form of jargon, mathematical equations whose relevance is obscure, peacock displays of name-dropping, misappropriation and misapplication of scientific theories are often seen in postmodernist 'discourse'. Nietzsche, Heidegger, Heisenberg, Einstein, Godel, Wittgenstein are hauled in and cited as saying things they didn't say . . .
>
> (Benson and Stangroom, 2006: 9)

Benson and Stangroom are highly critical of a general intellectual laziness which leads to truth not being sought, and being ignored or bastardised by religious fundamentalists and postmodernists. For Benson and Stangroom, not all opinions concerning the social and natural world are equal, and science has a long pedigree of truth-seeking. Facts exist and cannot be open to other interpretations. They cite the murder of millions throughout history in the many instances of massacres, war crimes, and ethnic cleansings.

However, from a realist perspective, murder *is* open to other interpretations. For example, humans killing humans can be categorised as criminal or legal, or morally justified or unwarranted, depending on how it is perceived. There is the intransitive reality of a dead body (or bodies) but the transitive event of killing can be considered in alternative ways (Morrall, 2006a). However, the realism I adhere to is never in denial about the 'workable' reality of the dead body whether from murder or malaria, nor about the associated pain and anguish.

SUMMARY

Theories are the sociologist's intellectual implements. For the stucturalist theorist, the individual exists within a social system, and that social system today is global-wide. The stucturalist not only theorises but also engineers. Society is regarded as containing structures that mould human performance and create opportunities for some, but adversities and inequalities for others. Therefore, social structures and perhaps (global) society overall has to be altered before, for example, disease can be contained and early death forestalled.

The interactionist sociologist plays down the influence of social structures and pays homage to the ability humans have as individuals to make their own meanings about their lives. Consequently, the interactionist people (as individuals and collectives) make up society, and have the potential to influence society rather than being the mere products of society. The profession of medicine has been exemplary in establishing meanings regarding human existence and in taking control of its own destiny as an occupational collective.

Constructionist sociology, and its extremist offspring, post-modernism, argues that there is an infinitive number of realities that can be organised by society or conjured up by humans. Nothing should be taken as actually factual (not even disease) but can be functionally factual (people experience disease as *dysfunctionally* real). People are at liberty to manufacture their own lifestyle, self-identity, and belief system, and thereby live as though there is a reality. Self-delusion is necessary to avoid the psychological terror of realising that nothing is essentially real and therefore nothing has any essential meaning.

The realist sociologist attempts to arbitrate between the other main sociological factions. For the realist, there really are facts (in nature and society), but these are frequently hidden by cultural meanings, symbols, and interpretations. So far, no system of investigative techniques (scientific or otherwise) has been able to expunge comprehensively the cultural coverings of all realities, although there are workable understandings for some presumed realities. As Simon Blackburn (2006) records, from Socrates onwards there has been a worthy search for truth by those sceptical enough to question what is on offer as truth. Medical science promises much more than it delivers in the way of truth because truths about health and disease remain obscure. However, truth, while perplexing, morally has to be searched for, not least because it may lead to reducing human suffering.

FURTHER READING

Giddens, A. (2006) *Sociology* (5th edn). Cambridge: Polity Press.
Ritzer, G. (2007) *Sociological Theory* (7th edn). Maidenhead: McGraw-Hill.

MORAL ACTION

Buy and read a 'thinking' journal/magazine (for example, *Prospect* magazine; *New Internationalist*; *Critical Public Health*) that you have not read previously, and surprise yourself with new ideas. If there aren't any new ideas, buy other magazines until you find your surprise.

HEALTH

2

D R THOMAS ALLINSON (1858–1918), English general practitioner and master baker, was struck off the medical register in 1892. What led to his medical defrocking were his ideas about how to be healthier. Ironically, many of his opinions on disease prevention are now official policy not only in England but throughout the Western world. Astoundingly, his ideas about the social significance of women's underwear are also of relevance in today's sexualising global society.

Living and working in Victorian London, when Britain was at its economic and political peak, Allinson was able to observe at close quarters the filth, squalor, and poverty of the many as well as the wealth and excesses of the few that characterised the first industrialised country.

Allinson believed that people were what they ate. What many people had as their daily diet at that time was rancid unwholesome food and polluted water which meant they were susceptible to disease and death at an average age of 43 years (Allinson, 2007; orig. 1893). He was against smoking when most medical practitioners in the nineteenth century either supported smoking or didn't regard it as harmful. He argued for daily exercise, and pointed out that over-eating and eating particular foods resulted in obesity. He found that drinking too much tea and coffee induced agitation and flatulence.

He didn't use alcohol and salt. He was a vegetarian, and an ardent advocate of whole-grain (wholemeal) bread. Prophetically, Allinson insisted that the trend towards a Western daily routine of bolting meals and engaging in little exercise because of the demands of work (although in his day many had manual jobs) was seriously detrimental to health.

Way ahead of his time on many personal and social issues, Allinson also tackled the problem of corsets, health, and feminism:

> The Lines of Nature cannot be improved by art. The fashion of drawing in the waist to make it look waspish, is both ungraceful and injurious. I look upon corsets as an evil invention, whereby a woman is lead to physical destruction. If women want to compete with a man on an equal footing, they must throw aside these things. I desire to see woman man's equal, able to hold her own, and not merely his slave. The more one considers, the more one will find that corsets have a great deal of ill health to answer for, as they cramp the figure and the mind, and help to make woman man's toy, instead of his equal, and helpmate.
>
> (Allinson, 2007; orig. 1893)

So, not only did this simple man-of-medicine identify the subjugation of women through sexual objectification seventy-seven years before the redoubtable Germaine Greer published *The Female Eunuch* (Greer, 1970), he foreran by nearly a century the policy of governments, NGOs, and his own profession, shifting from 'disease' to 'health'.

But what is health? Is a person healthy if he/she unknowingly has a tumour growing internally but regularly runs a marathon? At what point does that person stop being a 'runner' and become a 'terminally ill patient'? If my general practitioner, on the basis of medical examination, informs me that I am healthy, but I 'feel' unwell, who is right? Can a low-caste child from the Indian subcontinent ever be described as healthy if she or he eats half the amount of food and lives for only two-thirds of the lifespan of a child born into a high-caste family? The lifespan of British citizens is now nearly double that of those living in Victorian Britain. If, as Allinson believed, the latter were unhealthy, does it follow logically that in a hundred years time, when the British will live longer still (unless they all succumb to the mess of global society), people today will be considered to have been unhealthy? What, therefore, are the objective, subjective, and social facets of health?

OBJECTIVE DISEASE

Until relatively recently, the overriding interpretation of 'healthiness' was the absence of bodily or mental afflictions that either caused suffering to the individual concerned, incapacity in her or his daily activities, or were distressful to that person's family or community. That is, health has been for centuries defined as the absence of disease.

Furthermore, part of this anti-disease interpretation of health centres on morality. Being unhealthy in both pre-industrial and modern societies carries with it an element of personal failure and a duty to become well (Blaxter, 1990). To be unwell is a sign of inadequate willpower, even when disease transmission routes are unaffected by the most self-disciplined of individuals – Olympic gymnasts still do contract influenza, and long-distance runners can have heart attacks.

To an extent, all unhealthy people become socially excluded either permanently (as with chronic diseases such as AIDS and schizophrenia) or temporarily (as with most acute conditions). However, increasingly in Western countries those who abstain from alcohol, cigarette smoking, unprotected sex, and high fat and sugary foods, have the moral edge. Indulging in these practices may attract social stigma, loss of employment, and possibly the withdrawal of disease-care services, if patients are viewed by medical practitioners to be deliberately exposing themselves to 'unnecessary' risk.

Tribal healers, shamans, and witchdoctors in pre-industrial societies aimed to make their 'patient' well by removing malevolent spirits. For example, the traditional healers of the African Azande would suck from the body of a sufferer the 'evil pellets' thought to have been introduced into that person through witchcraft (Evans-Pritchard, 1937). Hippocrates (*c.* 460–*c.* 377 BC), using an approach that had its roots in ancient China and India, advocated the redressing of the balance between the four 'humours'. It was thought that these humours (black bile, yellow bile, blood, phlegm) were the essential constituents of the human body, and when in equilibrium a person was healthy, but when the balance was disturbed, then pain and disease ensued.

The ancient Greeks, of course, did not have the benefit of X-rays, scanning technology, or electron microscopes. Neither did they indulge in the surgical examination of either the living or the dead in a search for pathology. Although the second-century physician Galen (129–c. 199) did study human anatomy, a comprehensive understanding of the workings of the body came much later. Dissecting human corpses became acceptable only in the sixteenth century, and it was not until the seventeenth century that the circulation of blood was outlined by the English royal physician, William Harvey (1578–1657).

Thomas Sydenham (1624–1689), a self-taught medical practitioner, was to formulate a taxonomy of diseases, delineating such conditions as syphilis, measles, gout, and dysentery. In doing so, he emphasised the objectivity of disease as being separate from the sufferer. That is, the trend had been since ancient times to regard the individual and her or his state of health/disease as integral, and to accept that there was essentially only one 'malady' that caused all symptoms. The implication from Sydenham's work was that people were susceptible to a variety of diseases, and that these could be described in detail, their origin found, and specific treatments offered.

Further objectification of disease occurred in the eighteenth and nineteenth centuries with the advent of a hospital system in Paris which was unprecedented in its size. This allowed for the easy observation and investigation of large numbers of patients. Moreover, the introduction into the French clinics of such apparatus as the stethoscope, invented by French physician René Laennec (1781–1826), contributed to medical practice looking deeper and deeper into the body for the causes and effects of diseases.

Michel Foucault (1973) uses the term *Le regard* (translated into English as 'the gaze') to describe the way in which particular groups in society view the world. Clinicians in the eighteenth and nineteenth centuries searched for the cause and effect of disease within the patient's (dead or alive) body. From then on, *Le regard* of the medical practitioner became focused on the minute workings of the body, and in doing so was to lead to more control and regulation over what was to be considered 'normal' anatomy and physiology, and behaviour.

While the stethoscope allowed the physician to search for specific signs of pathological change in the functioning of the lungs and heart in France, in Germany progress had been made in the operation of the microscope, devised originally in the eighteenth century. This led to further explanatory 'reductionism' as now individual cells could be observed, and conceived of as the building-blocks of human (and animal) life.

It was Rudolf Virchow (1812–1902) who then was to make the connection between changes in the composition and performance of cells and the existence of certain diseases. The effect of micro-organisms such as bacteria on tissues and cells was discovered by French chemist and biologist Louis Pasteur (1822–1895) and the German scientist Robert Koch (1843–1910). These developments formed the foundation of scientific medicine.

However, whether healthiness is viewed as being obtained through the calming of generalised disturbances, the excision of renegade spirits, or the curing of identifiable and localised rogue cells and microscopic pathogens, there has been a focus on 'malfunction'. The shift from anti-disease to pro-health as philosophy and policy for Western governments and medical practitioners did not come about until the twentieth century (as the treatment of Dr Allinson in the nineteenth century by the medical establishment testifies). It was the World Health Organization's optimistically comprehensive definition of health that signified a global shift:

> . . . a state of complete physical, mental and social well-being and not merely the absence of disease or infirmity . . .
>
> (WHO, 1946)

Moreover, the WHO supported pro-health in its 'Health For All' Alma Ata declaration in 1977, in which all member countries were entrusted to attain its capacious ideal (WHO, 1978).

But rather than a complete shift, Western governments today tend to give attention to both disease-orientated and pro-health definitions. Consequently, there is confusion over which is being addressed and which service should be used. For example, the vast majority of consultations carried out by general practitioners concern the presentation by patients of signs and symptoms from established ailments. Yet general practitioner surgeries are expected to be at the forefront of primary care and preventative medicine. Despite the rhetoric of health promotion from politicians and practitioners, most of the health budget is spent on curative medicine. Both pro-health and anti-disease advice and policies continue (in their thousands) to come from the WHO and the multitude of other NGOs in the field of health/disease.

René Dubos (1979) points to the fallacy of health as an ideal state. He argues that the idea of perfect contentment has been projected by many cultures throughout history. He refers, for example, to the ancient Greeks whose legends cited tribes living in distant parts of the world in blissful conditions, not working and not suffering from disease or infirmity. With reference to later civilisations, Dubos observes that the eighteenth-century philosopher Jean-Jacques Rousseau (1712–1778) believed that the nearer humans were to nature, the healthier and happier they were. That is, Rousseau believed that humans became increasingly corrupted, both physically and mentally, the more 'civilised' they became.

Today, a 'happiness industry' has been created comprising of a disparate array of health-related faiths, including new-age philosophies, homeopathic potions, herbal remedies, 'holistic' doctrines, and bliss-inducing psychotherapies (Morrall, 2008a; 2008b). Although very different from each other in terms of their attestations and techniques, all have the intention of combating the destabilising effects of modern-day life, achieving mind–body harmony in one way or another, and getting closer to nature.

But for Dubos, this search for a state of equilibrium between humans and the natural world is based on a false premise. A few people may, perhaps with the assistance of secular or religious indoctrination, mind-pacifying drugs such as alcohol and marijuana, or mood-improving medication such as Prozac, be temporarily at ease with nature. However, most people for the majority of the time are ill-at-ease with nature. Nature is not a constant, resolute, or benign entity. Furthermore, the delimitation of 'natural' events and phenomena from 'unnatural' on the basis that the latter refers to human activity and the former everything else is erroneous.

For example, before humans even came on the scene in the world supposedly beginning the process of disrupting nature, the dinosaurs stomped around obliterating huge swathes of vegetation, killing other animals, or being prey to larger dinosaurs. Moreover, very suddenly they were wiped out by a cataclysmic event, quite probably involving meteors hitting the earth with such force that the resultant dust clouds thrown up into the atmosphere blocked out the sun's rays. Are these happenings any more 'natural' than the destruction of rainforests by South American and Tasmanian loggers, the killing of innocent civilians by the soldiers of countless numbers of countries, or the destruction of the ozone layer through the release into the atmosphere of chlorofluorocarbons (CFCs)?

Furthermore, what is a 'natural' environment for humans? Is it the arctic wastelands? Could it be the 'red centre' of the Australian outback? Might it be the sunny beaches of a Caribbean island? Or are vibrant and well-serviced cities not more natural habitats for humans, as well as for a plethora of animal life and vegetation? For sure, the natural environment throughout the world is changing – rapidly. James Lovelock (2007) and Fred Pearce (2006) argue that nature is about to take revenge on humanity because of the eco-logical damage it has caused. The tipping point towards climatic turbulence has been reached, and therefore humanity will either be exterminated or humans will have to come to terms with uncontrollable environments.

Moreover, there is a tension between individual happiness (in the sense of expressed and satisfied desires) and the common good. That is, the health of the individual may have to be sacrificed for the benefit of the health of society. Therefore, as Sigmund Freud (1930) was to argue, the basic ontological unease that humans have living in society can be seen as the consequence of successful social ties. For society to operate effectively, it is necessary to control aggressive and libidinous drives. This control, while having benefits for the individual (for example, to provide security), does produce negative consequences. Specifically, for Freud 'guilt' was an internalised mechanism generated by the moral standpoint of a particular culture in order to diminish the possibility of destructive (for society) hedonism. Freud's recognition of the interplay between society and the psyche is confirmation that he can be considered both as a psychologist and a sociologist (Bocock, 1976).

Dubos argues also that the search by the profession of medicine for specific cures to specific diseases is based on another false premise. He suggests that the profession of medicine's quest to find solutions for all diseases is a 'hopeless pursuit' because most conditions are caused by a multitude of factors. Symptoms may be controlled, but, apart from for a few notable exceptions (for example, smallpox), medicine has failed to rid the world of most of the diseases it has been able to categorise. Moreover, even those it has previously controlled may not always remain dormant (for example, tuberculosis).

Significantly, Dubos records that it was the very man who was to be so influential in the formulation of microbiological explanations of disease, Rudolf Virchow, who also recognised social factors in the creation of epidemics. Virchow was not only a scientist but also a social reformer who campaigned for action to be taken against poverty and overcrowding in order to prevent the spread of disease. Most infectious diseases have been made less virulent and less widespread through alterations to the social circumstances in which people live (better housing, safer working conditions, improved wages to buy more food), and sanitation and water supply, than by medical intervention. Medical practitioners, therefore, should provide individual treatment and support social change. This is the basis of much of the sociological critique of biomedicine, and also the basis of 'social medicine'.

For Dubos, health is not contingent solely on biological and psychological qualities. Taking a relativist position, Dubos argues that true health is where an individual believes herself or himself to be healthy, and is viewed as such by her or his social group. There is not, therefore, a universally applicable state of healthiness. It is, implies Dubos, the very spirit of humanity, characterised by a never-ending search for excitement, acquisition, and invention, that yields discontent. That is, a state of 'complete well-being' is unnatural for humans.

In order to substantiate the defining health as the absence of disease (that is, negatively) it has to be demonstrated that there are standard and universally applicable rules of human anatomy and physiology. That is, before we can know what is abnormal, there has to be a concrete understanding of normality. For example, we cannot possibly diagnose someone's blood pressure as too high if there is not an accurate measurement of what it should be in the first place. To know that a cell is growing in a malignant fashion, there must initially be an exact appreciation of how a cell grows usually.

A precise appreciation of the functioning of the liver must precede the deduction that a patient has cirrhosis.

However, there are no such guarantees of knowledge in all (and postmodernists argue, in any) areas of medical practice. Not only are there considerable uncertainties about what is normal and therefore what is abnormal, but the boundaries of the human body and mind are unclear and alter over time and place (Helman, 2007; Shilling, 2007).

In some cultures humans are physically delineated but are intertwined with others in their community and possibly with their dead relatives (who are hence not considered to be dead but very much alive in the members of the families who are less corporeally challenged). Ideas change from person to person about whether or not bodily fluids, hair, external genitalia, and previously held personal opinions and former personality traits are connected to or separate from the 'real' him/her. If they are part of him/her are they permanent or temporary?

Moreover, where are the borders of the body and mind in consumer society and in cyberspace? If an individual's lifestyle and self-identity is heavily or totally influenced by the commodities he/she procures, then does that person not also become a pastiche of those commodities or perhaps a supra-commodity (a combination of inanimate and animate elements forming an entity beyond the sum of its parts)?

SUBJECTIVE ILLNESS

While health can be defined either as an ideal state or the absence of disease (and disease is what doctors describe), illness is the subjective experience of 'feeling' unwell:

> *Illness* can be taken to mean the experiences of disease, including the feelings relating to changes in bodily states and the consequences of having to bear that ailment; illness, therefore, relates to a way of being for the *individual concerned*.
>
> (Radley, 1994: 3; emphases in the original)

Illness, therefore, is what the individual senses that is 'wrong' with her or him, and may lead to making an appointment to see a doctor.

Disease is what the individual has wrong with her or him on the return from that appointment.

For Cecil Helman (2007), a wide variety of subjective evidence is involved in the process of defining oneself as ill. These perceived alterations can be in physiognomy (for example, loss or gain of weight), bodily emissions (for example, urinating frequently, or diarrhoea), the working of specific organs (for example, heart beating fast, or headaches), or the emotions (for example, depression, or anxiety).

However, whether or not an illness is experienced in the first place, what meaning in attached to any pain or discomfort, the reaction the individual has to her or his illness, and the way in which both healers and society frame and respond to the individual, are all dependent upon the social context in which events are taking place:

> One cannot really understand how people react to illness, death or other misfortunes without an understanding of the type of culture they have grown up in or acquired – that is, of the 'lens' through which they perceive and interpret their world. In addition it is also necessary to examine the *social organisation* of health and illness in that society (the healthcare system), which includes the ways in which people have become recognized as ill, the ways that they present this illness to other people, the attributes of those they present their illness to, and the ways that illness is dealt with.
>
> (Helman, 2007: 7)

A ten-point inventory of reasons why people proceed from feeling ill towards being diagnosed as diseased was formulated in the 1960s by David Mechanic, a founder of sociological analysis of health/ disease. Mechanic realised that there are many psychological and social phases before a person is diagnosed as suffering from an 'objective' medical condition. For Mechanic (1968) the factors affecting an individual seeking help from a medical practitioner will depend on whether on not symptoms:

(a) are highly visible and recognisable;
(b) are regarded as serious/dangerous;
(c) disrupt family and working responsibilities and other social routines;
(d) repeat or persist;

(e) breach the sufferer's tolerance level and/or that of others;
(f) are understood well in terms of cause, treatment, and prognosis;
(g) are feared greatly or feared only minimally (leading in either case to denial and avoidance or medical help being sought);
(h) figure high in the individual's hierarchy of needs when compared with other priorities;
(i) are interpreted as with other 'normal' activities (such as long working hours, bereavement, or physical exertion) rather than disease.
(j) can be treated easily in terms of available resources and time, and without embarrassment.

Many if not all of these factors continue to apply. For example, it is well documented that visits to general practitioners are influenced by gender-role performance and employment responsibilities (Nettleton, 2006).

The process of becoming a patient (that is, the individual's social status moving from 'feeling ill' to 'being diseased') is not only dependent on the beliefs and actions of the individual, which in themselves are affected by social factors, but also upon the behaviour of disease-care practitioners. In my study of how people became the patients of mental health professions (Morrall, 1998) I recorded how community psychiatric nurses (CPNs) act as gatekeepers for the psychiatric services. CPNs make decisions to attend general practitioners' surgeries on the basis of whether or not they need 'extra' patients on their caseloads, or at times to ensure that they retain good relationships with medical colleagues by taking 'difficult' patients off their hands. In doing so, they are regulating who does and who doesn't begin (or continue) a career as a mentally 'diseased' patient.

In the shaping of her or his recognition and appreciation of illness, the individual is interacting with her or his environment and significant others. Seeking medical help becomes merely one possible response to illness. In the vast majority of cases, however, medical attention is not sought when a person feels ill. That is, most illness is dealt with by the individual herself or himself without any recourse to formal help from doctors or other disease-care workers. A high proportion of the population has been reported as suffering from symptoms of illnesses that are not reported to medical practitioners. However, people may also suffer very debilitating symptoms (particularly mental problems) without attending a doctor's surgery (Cockerham, 2007). This difference between the incidence and the prevalence of disease can be described as the 'health iceberg' (that is, only a small percentage of the overall illness experienced by people is officially detailed), although 'disease iceberg' is a more accurate term.

The term 'sickness' denotes the amalgamation of the two processes of feeling ill and being diagnosed as diseased. It alludes to the existence of a social role especially following a diagnosis, and that there are obligations and rights that society confers on diseased individuals (as well as on the disciplines of disease).

The WHO interpretation of health, as Aubrey Lewis (1953) has suggested, is so all-encompassing and idealistic that it is worthless in any pragmatic sense. Moreover, those advocating such a definition miss the point that for most of the time both doctors and lay people do conceptualise health as the absence of disease.

For Lewis, an individual's belief that she or he is in good health (because he/she experiences no pain, discomfort, or loss of function), is, of course, in marked contrast to the physician's scientific diagnosis of disease using, for example, the stethoscope, microbiological analysis, or, today, complex scanning technology. The subjective vindication for feeling healthy is accomplished through the unconscious or conscious device of inspecting one's body and mind for malfunctioning and discomfort. The objective approach is to use medical technology and knowledge to confirm or refute the actuality of ailments and injuries.

However, medical and lay beliefs are not necessarily dichotomous ways of understanding disease/health. In most medical examinations, the patient's account of her or his illness is obtained and incorporated into the process of diagnosing disease. Realistically, the doctor and the patient negotiate their respective perceptual territories, objectively and subjectively colluding to reach a diagnostic conclusion, which then may be redefined by the patient on leaving the surgery or by a medical specialist if further investigations are sought.

For Alan Radley (1994) the negotiation between medical practitioners and patients over the meaning of health/disease foments what he calls the 'therapeutic illusion'. That is, ostensibly there is an acceptance (no matter how tenuous or contrived) of the efficacy of medical science by patients and doctors. Where non-compliance (on behalf of the patient) occurs, this is as a result of an unresolvable clash between the subjective and objective accounts. The exceptions (that is, when no negotiation can take place) are when an individual is unconscious as a result of an accident, or during surgery. Moreover, an individual's disquiet about, for example, a constant feeling of tiredness would in one way or another have been influenced by medical discourse which links lethargy to such conditions as iron-deficiency anaemia or seasonal affective disorder. The person concerned may have read about the link between her/his symptom in popular magazines, watched a television programme containing details of new medical approaches in these areas, or downloaded copious amounts of information (both credible and dubious) from the Internet.

Individuals themselves may have quite irreconcilable and fluctuating beliefs, which may be connected to his/her gender, ethnicity, economic class, or age. For example, the same person may have a fatalistic attitude towards lung cancer and continue to smoke, as well as producing a 'fat-file' by attending frequently his/her general practitioner's surgery over what appear to be trivial medical complaints. That individual's conceptualisation of his/her ailments may also fluctuate between orthodox, complementary/alternative, and folk explanations. Moreover, for one person the loss of a limb or a diagnosis of a fatal disease may be experienced as a personal health disaster, whereas for another it may spur him/her to achieve incredible physical feats which most 'healthy' people could not accomplish:

> Terminal cancer sufferer Jane Tomlinson died aged 43 in 2007, following a seven-year battle with the disease. The married mother-of-three, who was made CBE for charitable services in June, had raised £1.75m in a series of gruelling challenges. Her last big challenge was a 6700km bike ride across America.
>
> (BBC Leeds, 2007)

Personal endeavours such as Tomlinson's cross the objective–subjective barrier. They also transcend the debilitating 'spoiled identity' brought about by stigmatising disease labels, and not only re-establish an 'untainted identity' but affirm a 'super-identity'.

SOCIAL SICKNESS

That there are social features in the maintenance of health and the manifestation of disease is irrefutable. This is the case whether health and disease are considered discernible entities (the positivist position of medical scientists and sociological structuralists) or fallacious phenomena conjured up by medical and political discourses (the stance taken by constructionist-/postmodernist-leaning social commentators).

Susan Sontag's (1990) constructionist-leaning historical analysis of disease shows how conditions with an unknown cause and ineffective treatment attract extraordinary levels of apprehension and disgust and/or romantic connotations. Sontag records that in the eighteenth century 'consumption' (pulmonary tuberculosis) became a symbol of gentility and vulnerability within the upper classes. Sufferers were viewed as having a 'sensitive' constitution. Internally, the disease was adorned as organic 'decor'. Externally, to appear 'consumptive' (pale and drained) was to be fashionable. To have the 'tubercular look' became a metaphor for exemplary breeding or a bohemian and artistic lifestyle.

By the mid-nineteenth century, however, with the discovery of the responsible germ, the same disease had acquired a fearful reputation as an insidious contagion, and indiscriminate killer of children and adults. Sufferers from the 'lower orders' in particular were considered to be morally and physically contagious, and consequently shunned by their communities. Cancer and AIDS were to replace tuberculosis as the mysterious, awesome, and repugnant diseases of the twentieth century.

While diseases can have metaphorical overtones, for the structuralist there is the unavoidable stark reality of disease.

Frederick Engels, Karl Marx's intellectual collaborator and financial supporter, wrote a social history of England's working classes in the winter of 1844–1845. He described the appalling social conditions experienced by the poor living in the large industrial cities of that age. He also connected the cause of morbidity and mortality among the inhabitants of the slum areas, factory workers, and the unemployed, to these social conditions. Engel's treatise is one of the earliest and richest accounts of how disease cannot be simply understood in terms of biology and pathology. In this extract Engels lays the blame for disease and death on the way in which (capitalist) society is structured, and in particular on the bourgeoisie:

> The manner in which the great multitude of the poor is treated by society today is revolting. They are drawn into large cities where they breathe a poorer atmosphere than in the country; they are relegated to districts which, by reasons of the method of construction, are worse ventilated than any others; they are deprived of all means of cleanliness, of water itself, since pipes are laid only when paid for, and the rivers are so polluted that they are useless for such purposes; they are obliged to throw all offal and garbage, all dirty water, often all disgusting drainage and excrement into the streets ... They are given damp dwellings, cellar dens that are not waterproof from below, or garrets that leak from above ... They are deprived of all enjoyments except that of sexual indulgences and drunkenness, are worked every day to the point of complete exhaustion ... How is it possible, under such conditions, for the lower class to be healthy and long-lived?
>
> (Engels, 1999; orig. 1892: 128–129)

The circumstances in which the poor of the nineteenth century lived might seem to be no longer of relevance to the situation those living and working in urban regions have to contend with in twenty-first-century Western cities. What Stephen Halliday (2008) refers to as 'The Great Filth' of Victorian cities does not any more characterise English cities or those of other post-industrial countries.

But small sections of many of today's Western cities, inhabited by a growing socially excluded underclass, do replicate the conditions of the Great Filth. Moreover, throughout global society vast numbers of people are living in filth caused by rapid and uncontrolled urbanisation and/or industrialisation (by 2008 the global urban population had overtaken the rural population).

A study conducted in the late 1990s of the Indian city of Mumbai recorded how the systematic clearance of slum areas for new commercial and residential developments was responsible for the eviction of 167,000 people (Emmel and D'Souza, 1999). One group of slum dwellers, who had been brought from their villages to work as labourers, were moved scores of times from their homes by demolition squads from land that had become valuable in the drive to modernise Mumbai. They now live in mangrove swamps reclaimed from the sea but which still become water logged at high tide.

The children of these slum dwellers have protracted nutritional deprivation, diarrhoea, respiratory disease, and skin infections, which were linked to the transitory nature of their residence and the effect this has on the family finances:

> Repeated eviction wears away at the household economy. Each time the huts were demolished, the women explained, money had to be found to rebuild the shelters . . . As one woman told us 'each time our hut is destroyed there is less money to feed the children. Who will feed the children?'
>
> (Emmel and D'Souza, 1999: 1118)

A government programme to rehouse these people into blocks of small apartments (paid for by the property tycoons building expensive accommodation on the former slum site), where there is a shortage of water, toilets, and effective household waste disposal, may lead merely to re-establishing the previous levels of filth for what had become a population of five million. Horizontal slums may become vertical slums (Giridharadas, 2006).

The emergence of the 'Second Great Filth' indicates (from a Marxist perspective) the most manifest of capitalism's contradictions – immense wealth existing alongside intense poverty. The wealth–poverty schism occurs throughout global society, including the richest country (the USA), and leads inexorably to another of capitalism's great contradictions: inequality of access to services.

For example, in 2007 a health insurance company (Cigna) refused to pay for 17-year-old Natalie Sarkisyan's life-saving liver transplant following complications from a bone marrow operation. The company's position was that the operation was experimental and therefore unproven. Her family could not afford to pay for the transplant ($75,000). Medical and nursing staff along with the girl's relatives conducted a protest outside the offices of the company. The company relented and offered to pay for the operation. Natalie Sarkisyan died a few hours later (Pilkington, 2007).

Added to the filth and contradictions is what the World Bank has admitted is a global food crisis caused by the great crisis of global warming (assisted by iniquitous international food production and trading arrangements, and latterly the crisis in the world's financial system), which could push a further 100 million people into extreme poverty (World Bank, 2008a; 2008b). The palpability of the filth, contradictions, and crises may exacerbate global social disorder (Brunelle, 2008). Potentially, the mess of global society could be indicative of the collapse of capitalism, albeit somewhat later than Marx had predicted.

Wild fluctuations in food prices and supplies are occurring at a time when advice about diet abounds. Echoing Dr Allinson's visionary proclamations, the message being disseminated throughout the world from governments and the WHO is that bad diets cause disease (whether by not eating the right food, eating the wrong food, eating too much food, or not eating enough food). Diet has always been prominent in human personal and social life. Humans (like all life sources) need nourishment to survive and (unlike most other life sources) as a significant part of their culture. But the difference today is that food has become thoroughly politicised.

Food production and distribution is a matter of politics and so, therefore, is what as individuals we eat to make us healthy or diseased because it is controlled by fiscal and tax policies, by the commercial interests of global corporations, by consumer lobby groups, as well as by personal choice (Robertson et al., 1999; Marshall, 2000; Nestle, 2007). For example, we as individuals may want to swallow a banquet of fat-laden, salt-laden, and sugar-laden processed comestibles (and doing so block our arteries and cause our heart to become ischaemic) but are faced with much admonishment from the 'health police'. However, counsel from governments and NGOs not to eat too much fat, salt, and sugar is not hugely persuasive when we are also subjected to bombardments of sophisticated sales techniques to encourage us to do the opposite.

As Marion Nestle (2007) demonstrates, food is an enormously lucrative industry and hence is hugely manipulative. The selling of bananas and beetroot does not make as much profit as burgers and biscuits. Furthermore, while politicians ostensibly are campaigning for people to become healthier, they are subjected to pressures from the food industry to curtail their enthusiasm for dietary change for at least as long as it takes for the industry to readjust and market 'healthy foods' at inflated prices.

But the most blatant attempts to undermine policies aimed at preventing serious disease have come from tobacco companies. Evidence of cigarette smoking being a source of lung cancer was available for a very long time before it was accepted by the tobacco companies. In many Western countries, legislation has been introduced to curb this killer commodity (public disease warnings; prohibition on smoking in the workplace, on public transport, and other public places). However, tobacco companies have since either exploited the black-market trade in cigarettes within the West or shifted their trade to the underdeveloped and developing parts of the world, thereby exporting the epidemic of cancer and ischaemia (Maguire and Campbell, 2000; Boyle *et al.*, 2004; Helman, 2007). For example, smoking is responsible for 930,000 premature deaths in India (Jha *et al.*, 2008).

Target countries are attempting to fight against tobacco companies. Nigeria, for example, has sought billions of dollars in damages through the courts for the allegedly cynical attempts by the companies to hook the young onto their products using sales techniques no longer legal in the West (McGreal, 2008b).

The connection between the economic success of a country and the concomitant development of its social infrastructure (such as welfare support, health/disease services, safety at work, and the management of environmental pollution) and health has been well documented. An important measurement of health/disease is life expectancy. Assessment of life expectancy can be made in two ways. Either the actual average life expectancy of a country can be used or this can be adjusted for the years spent in good/poor health.

Using the latter method (which is favoured by the WHO), the British Economic and Social Research Council (ESRC) reports on global differences. In Britain it is 70.6 years, in Japan it is 75 years, and in Russia 59 years (dropping from 65 years since the break-up of the USSR), whereas in Sierra Leone it is less than 29 years (ESRC, 2008). It is not just how early people die that depends on where in the world they live, but from what they will die. Heart disease, strokes, and cancer are bigger killers in rich countries, and infectious diseases (including HIV/AIDS, malaria, tuberculosis, and the emerging infectious disease such as eboli and severe acute respiratory virus) kill more in poor countries (ESRC, 2008; Jones *et al.*, 2008).

Children's life expectancy is also dependent on the socio-economic status of their country. As with life expectancy overall, there has been a significant improvement in child survival globally. However, the divergence is immense. Whereas there are six deaths before the age of five per live 1,000 births in most developed countries (with only three in Sweden, Singapore, San Marino, Liechtenstein, Iceland and Andorra), Sierra Leone has 270 deaths before the age of five per 1,000 live births, Angola, 260, Afghanistan, 257, Niger, 253, and Liberia, 235. Every day 26,000 children under five die mostly from diseases that can be prevented through vaccination, better nutrition, safe water, better sanitation and hygiene, or basic medical input (United Nations Children's Fund, 2008).

The relationship between socio-economic inequalities and disease inequalities within rich countries is reified in the life expectancy figures with those at the bottom of the socio-economic hierarchy dying younger than those at the top, children born into families of low socio-economic status having a much higher risk of death before five years of age.

Moreover, differences in disease-care provision and access can also be enormous between developed countries. The experience of British journalist Alan Wilkinson (1997) of becoming ill when visiting New York is illuminating. The USA has minimal 'free' provision supplied in its public hospitals. Although carrying holiday insurance, he went to the local public hospital as he had difficulty in breathing, and was (eventually) diagnosed as having pneumonia. Apart from the not unexpected wait in a crowed casualty department for four hours, and the highly predictable indignity of being asked what language the English speak by the registration attendant, he found that he was the only white patient. A further extensive wait of five hours for a bed gave him the opportunity to observe closely his fellow patients and the actions of the medical staff:

> There was a junkie, collapsed across two chairs. There was the woman with the blood-soaked leg. 'That mother-f*****! I shoulda killed him', she groaned. There was the hero on crutches, grimacing manfully. 'Hey, it's where the bullet lodged, man. Kinda pus and blood oozing out, right?'. And then there was the demented, neglected, rotting poor. A Hispanic woman wrapped in a bathrobe.

'Ees my legs doctor'. He gestured with his stethoscope. There were no concessions to modesty. Just 'Open Up' . . . A morose Nicaraguan peeled off a sock to reveal a rotten foot almost split in two. The doctor asked a colleague if he thought it was safe to touch it. The consensus was he'd better not: give the guy a jar of Vitamin E jelly and get him out.

(Wilkinson, 1997)

Despite spending more than any other country in the world on disease care, there may be as many as one in three citizens of the USA who do not have any or adequate health insurance. Therefore, nearly 100 million people have to use the public system which continues to be deeply flawed because of chaotic administration and chronic underfunding (Families USA, 2007).

The British public disease-care system, the National Health Service (NHS), was set up in 1946 by the post-Second World War Labour Government. The explicit mandate the government set the NHS was to harmonise the health/disease status of people at the lower end of the social scale with that found among people at the top. But it has failed. Overall, morbidity and mortality rates within all British social groups have improved, but the setting up of the NHS to reduce disease inequalities has had the paradoxical effect of making people further down the social hierarchy more, not less diseased when compared with those at the top.

The seminal 'Black Report' published in 1980 reported on disease inequalities in Britain (Townsend et al., 1992). It concluded that, at all stages of life, people belonging to the lower socio-economic groups had comparatively worse health than those in the top groups. The specific observations of the Black Report were:

(a) There are marked differences in mortality rates between the occupational groups, for both sexes, and in all age groups.

(b) Twice as many babies born to unskilled manual parents die within the first month of life compared to babies born to parents in the professional occupational class.

(c) Approximately three times as many infants born to unskilled manual parents die within the first year of life compared to babies born to parents in the professional occupational class.

(d) Rates of self-reported chronic illness are twice as high among men in the unskilled occupational class compared to men in the professional occupational class.

(e) Rates of self-reported chronic illness are two and a half times as high among wives of men in the unskilled occupational class compared to wives of men in the professional occupational class.

(f) Men and women from the unskilled manual occupational class are two and a half times more likely to die before reaching the age of retirement compared to men and women in the professional occupational class.

Crucially, the Black Report gave notification that the NHS could not in any dramatic way alter these disease inequalities. The key social (rather than health/disease) issues were – and still are – unemployment, lack of decent education, shoddy housing, and inadequate transport to connect people with essential services such as shops and medical facilities. The tenor of the thirty-seven recommendations made in the Black Report was that, in order to reduce disease inequalities, there had to be a major increase in public expenditure to improve working and living conditions. That is, to tackle disease and premature death effectively within one country (Britain), social inequalities have to be addressed structurally. By extension, the structure of global society needs to be altered to reduce disease inequalities between countries.

Other explanations for inequalities in disease besides that of the structuralist position have been well rehearsed (Townsend *et al.*, 1992; Davey and Seale, 1996; Nettleton, 2006). For example, from an interactionist perspective, people make meaningful choices about how to conduct their lives. An individual's decision to smoke, overindulge in alcohol, take little physical exercise, and eat high fatty, salty, sugary foods has been made action because it has meaning for him/her. He/she has not been compelled to eat a pizza, drink a bottle of vodka, followed by a bowl of ice cream and a cigarette while sitting in front of the television. It is not the result of explicit coercion or subliminal direction by the owners of the industries selling these products, their advertising agents, and the hegemony of free-market politics. People have a choice as to whether or not, as Dr Allinson recommended, they eat healthy food, take exercise, and don't smoke (and release their corsets).

Moreover, the individual's micro and macro cultural affiliations and interactions may be sufficiently cogent to reduce the effects of structural pressures. Through daily interaction with friends, family, working colleagues, and the surrounding community, the individual is likely to have her or his behaviour modified. It is far easier to maintain a healthy eating and exercise regime if one's partner, peers, and business associates are like-minded. Equally, if an individual's interactions are with groups that have norms associated with drugs and lethargy, then the chances are that he/she will follow suit.

The 'social selection' perspective suggests that social class is viewed as the outcome of an involuntary and evolutionarily determined sorting process that is 'normal' for human populations. It is argued from this paradigm that some people are genetically more physically and mentally capable than others, and this will result inevitably in a rank order based on how fit a person is in the evolutionary race to survive. These innate biological and psychological characteristics mean that some individuals are born to have bad health and to die early, and the same group will be social underachievers. Hence, the lower social classes (those with meagre employment and educational, and material deprivation) contain most of the unhealthy people in society, not because of any causal relationship between the two, as is propounded by both the structuralists and the interactionsists, but because they 'naturally' occur together. Those with physical and mental disease will 'drift' into the disadvantaged stratum of society as a matter of course. The physically and mentally advantaged will maintain good health and gain social superiority. Self-evidently, the uneducated and unemployed, living in poor housing within disruptive communities, are more likely to be ill than are people with high educational and occupational attainment living in expensive and gated residential areas.

However, not only is this simplistic social selection theorising morally bankrupt (the danger is that if accepted, then nothing needs to be or can be done to alter disease inequalities), but the evidence is weak. Intergenerational social mobility is far more dependent on educational, cultural, and material factors than on health/disease. That is, it is much more probable that where a family values educational attainment and is financially assured, any progeny will either be as successful as the parents, or be propelled into a higher class, than any illness present causing a downward spiral. As far as intragenerational movement is concerned, if serious illness occurs in childhood, then this can effect social mobility. Long-term conditions such as respiratory disease and schizophrenia, if contracted at an early age, may produce a drift down the social scale, but the number affected in this way only accounts for a small proportion of those who are ill and indigent.

Furthermore, while organic and evolutionary drives may play their part in shaping behaviour, these would logically not push the individual in the direction of self-destruction. That is, swallowing large numbers of hamburgers, drinking copious amounts of alcohol, habitual smoking of cigarettes, and avoiding any physical exertion beyond walking to a bar or tobacconist, is not compatible with biological survival. Whatever biogenetic imperatives there are in human behaviour, these are patently overridden by the effects of cultural interactions and social structures with respect to disease inequalities.

A classic longitudinal research study deserves special mention in the debate about the relevance of the structuralist perspective. This is the 'Whitehall Study'. Michael Marmot and his colleagues (Marmot et al., 1984) carried out an analysis of the health/disease status of 17,000 male civil servants based in London over many years, starting at the end of the 1960s. At the beginning of the study the civil servants were examined medically to provide a baseline of their health/disease. After seven years, more than one thousand had died, with the cause of death, heart disease, found in half of the cases. However, there were higher death rates among the lower grades of workers compared to those with senior positions, with the death-rate gradient being proportionate to each tier of seniority. The lower grades of civil servants had almost four times the death rate of the very top civil servants.

What the Whitehall study has indicated is that the hierarchy of workplace organisations corresponds to the health/disease status of employees. Evidence from this study, therefore, implies that relative deprivation rather than absolute deprivation is the significant determinant of morbidity and mortality. Furthermore, even when no detectable disease was discernible at the start of the study, the lower the grade of the employee, the higher the death rate. That is, any recruitment of diseased civil servants to work in unskilled roles could not account for the mortality rate in this group.

Marmot *et al.* (1984) have demonstrated that occupational status is a robust predictor of such life-threatening conditions. Certain work-based psychosocial factors, such as autonomy and variety or direction and monotony, as experienced by employees, appeared to be critical for good or bad health. A major insight from the study was that both men and women in lower civil service grades reported that they had less control over their work, were given repetitive and unskilled tasks, and had a slower pace of work, compared with those in higher grades, and that job satisfaction was correspondingly lower. Absence from work because of sickness was coupled to occupational grade and perceptions of job satisfaction. Whether measuring short periods of absence (that is, under seven days) or longer terms (seven days or over), dissatisfied lower-grade employees were much more likely to be off work. The most unhappy employees in the lowest ranks had up to six times the rate of sickness as the most high-ranking and content employees.

The Whitehall Study was continued for over twenty years. Aided by the conclusions from a range of European and Australasian research, it has established clearly the relationship between position in the social hierarchy and morbidity and mortality. Social gradient not only affects how long a person can expect to live, but whether or not he/she is likely to contract heart disease, some cancers, chronic lung disease, gastrointestinal disease, depression, suicide, 'stress', back pain, generally feeling unwell, and hence how much sick leave will be taken (Ferrie, 2004). Furthermore, the Whitehall researchers state that any health promotion policy reliant on exhorting individuals to change their performance (that is, telling people how to eat, drink, exercise, and to stop smoking) is inadequate because what is required is altering the structural refashioning of work and other aspects of social life.

Sir Michael Marmot, Professor of Epidemiology and Public Health (and now Director of the International Institute for Society and Health at University College London, and Chair of the WHO Commission on Social Determinants of Health), explains the interplay between structural conditions and health/disease:

[I]f you are a fifteen-year-old boy in Lesotho, your chance of reaching the age of 60 is about 10 per cent. If you are a fifteen-year-old boy in Sweden, your chance of reaching 60 is 91 per cent.

This difference is due to social conditions, which are determinants of health. They include education and the nature of jobs. They include living conditions such as housing and availability of adequate nutritious food. They also entail access to quality healthcare.

Similarly, there are big health inequalities within countries. Let's take the United States, for example. If you catch the metro train in downtown Washington, D.C., to suburbs in Maryland, life expectancy is 57 years at beginning of the journey. At the end of the journey, it is 77 years. This means that there is [a] 20-year life expectancy [disparity] in the nation's capital, between the poor and predominantly African American people who live downtown, and the richer and predominantly non-African American people who live in the suburbs.

(Marmot, 2008)

Marmot also observes that being poor in inner-city Washington, D.C. is a different experience from being poor in Lesotho, but what both have in common is the lack of control that people have over their respective lives and over their physical environments.

Richard Wilkinson (1999; 2006), Professor of Medical Epidemiology at the University of Nottingham, UK, also accepts that the solution to disease inequalities lies in attacking the structural determinants of the social environment. However, he does not believe that this means that economic growth should be relied on to provide better circumstances for the poor in the developed countries and for people in the underdeveloped/developing parts of the world. He points out that improved economic performance may have a 'trickle-down' effect on social disadvantage. That is, those at the bottom of the social hierarchy benefit from the conspicuous consumption of those at the top due to, for example, the consequential increased employment. However, this, suggests Wilkinson, will only serve to reinforce the differences in material wealth/poverty and health/disease between social groups. It may also bring global ecological disaster.

Wilkinson argues that the overall burden on society and the developing world of disadvantage needs to be addressed through the implementation of policies on employment, income, and education. These policies must be aimed at altering the structural conditions that in turn foment social determinants of disease and premature death. He speculates that it is specifically income inequality that leads to a loss of a sense of dignity, self-respect, and confidence. This then results in the atrophication of social relationships, which reduces further the individual's ability to cope with everyday life events. It is plausible, suggests Wilkinson, that these feelings of inferiority will induce chronic anxiety and thereby make the individual far more prone to infectious and cardiovascular diseases than if he/she was valued by society.

This approach, posits Wilkinson, helps to account for the concurrence of low social status, fragile or non-existent social networks, chronic anxiety, and serious disease. Moreover, prolonged exposure to personal and social difficulties will reduce an individual's 'health capital' (his/her innate and acquired reserve of healthiness) and exacerbate biological predilection to disease. That is, an individual's 'life course' becomes imbedded into his/her physiology and can fuel pathology (Blane, 1999; Davey-Smith, 2003).

Wilkinson provides an example of the inadequacy of the 'individualistic' approach to disease inequalities. He observes that there is already a public awareness of the disease risks associated with an inadequate and unwholesome diet, and inactivity (much more than Dr Allinson could have dreamed of). Political endeavour, therefore, needs not to be directed any more at the individual to eat healthily and jog more frequently, but at the food manufacturers who promote fatty beefburgers and highly sweetened drinks aimed at children, and salt-ridden processed ready-made meals at adults.

Furthermore, the cost of healthy food is usually more than that of unhealthy food. Consequently, a remedy could be for government to install fiscal incentives that would redress this imbalance and enable those families on low wages or who are unemployed to make their choice of diet go beyond the consumption of cheap calories. As Wilkinson notes, foods and drinks soaked in sugar, fat, and salt may be eaten 'for comfort' when people do not have lifestyle alternatives due to their material circumstances, and lack of educational and employment scope. Comfort foods, alcohol, and smoking provide a temporary escape from social oppression and personal despondency.

SUMMARY

Human health is an incongruous concept. Medical science objectifies health as what is left (biologically and psychologically) when disease is not present. Individuals experience health subjectively, and while they partake in the process of medical objectification, their 'illness' may not confer with the doctor's diagnosis of 'disease'.

This mismatch is being aggravated on the one side by medicine and most of the other disciplines of disease espousing the need to substantiate their practices with 'evidence' and utilising technology for diagnosis and treatment; on the other side, by people turning to and being drawn in by, the prolific and profitable alternative/complementary therapy industry. Further ambiguity is heaped on the concept of health when people are objectively wracked with disease but feel healthy and seek neither medical nor complementary/alternative help, or are objectively disease-free and insist on receiving the services of either or both.

Moreover, as Helman (2007) so capably explains, the culture to which an individual belongs determines the degree to which biological and psychological states are considered healthy or diseased. But, notwithstanding these subjective and cultural considerations, Helman does not falter in his appreciation that disease really does exist and causes real human suffering, and that sickness is created by society:

> *poverty* may result in poor nutrition, overcrowded living conditions, inadequate clothing, low levels of education, housing (or work) sited in areas with greater environmental dangers (such as near factories producing toxic chemicals), as well as exposure to physical and psychological violence, psychological stress, and drug and alcohol abuse.
>
> (Helman, 2007: 5; emphasis in the original)

The link between social inequalities and disease inequalities (within and between countries) is so obvious, and has been so well researched that it is accepted by most social scientists and policy-makers. Generally accepted also is the widening of social inequality. It follows that, as global social inequalities are widening, then so are disease inequalities.

Appreciating the effects of (global) society on health/disease has the corollary that society must be transformed if the health of all of humanity is to be improved to the level that has been achieved by the socially privileged or to a height that has yet to be reached by any social group. As Marmot (2008) argues, global *action* is required to address the social determinants of health/disease.

In part, this action is about doctors, nurses, and the other disease practitioners carrying out their normal work wherever they are located (cleanly, kindly, and competently). However, it is also about them fulfilling their moral responsibilities for global health/disease. Without this wider social campaigning dimension their labours are, in respect of the totality of disease, ineffectual and immoral.

Helman is a culturally sensitive socially aware medical practitioner, and I (respectfully) suggest a closet realist. That is, his de facto realism materialises from his understanding that there is truth hidden inside the cultural packaging of social and physical phenomena. Helman also practices what he preaches, as his fascinating autobiographical account of his career as a general practitioner in London, *Suburban Shaman: Tales from Medicine's Frontline*, testifies (Helman, 2006).

Dr Allinson was no mental masturbator either. His social campaigning challenged medical and political orthodoxy, and his nineteenth-century dictums on health, so very familiar in the twenty-first century, were put into practice, and 'Allinson Wholemeal Bread' is still sold (although his original company is now part of a colossal global corporation).

However, Allinson's diatribe on evil underwear (attacking its deleterious effect on the female form and liberation), has not been so predictive. Indeed, even the redoubtable Greer, although aware, like Allinson, of the symbolic connotations of the corset, failed to predict the extent to which her eunuch would figuratively and literally become 'basqued'. In 2008 my Internet search (using Google) produced nearly five million hits for 'corset'.

FURTHER READING

Dubos, R. (1979) *Mirage of Health*. New York: Harper Colophan.

MORAL ACTION

Join, and be active in, a human rights organisation (such as Amnesty International or Human Rights Watch; Save The Children; Physicians For Human Rights).

SCIENCE

3

> In the sphere of thought, sober civilisation is roughly synonymous
> with science. But science unadulterated, is not satisfying; men [and
> women] need also passion and art and religion. Science may set
> limits to knowledge, but should not set limits to imagination.
>
> (Bertrand Russell, 1961: 36)

SCIENCE HAS BEEN STEADILY EXPROPRIATED by the medical
profession over hundreds of years to support its premises and
procedures, and to further its occupational status.

Most of the other disease disciplines have followed medicine's
lead in espousing a scientific justification for their role and
prestige. Whether it's nursing, midwifery, occupational therapy,
physiotherapy, or audiology, science (in the guise of 'evidence-
based practice') has been commandeered to legitimise knowledge
and practice.

But what is science? Is science separate to passion, art, and religion? Is the application of science to disease-care realisable?

Scientific thought has become the prevailing and most imposing
epistemology in the West and through globalisation that of the
world. However, sociological thinking has challenged the authenticity and authority of science. An obvious observation is that

superstition, religion, folklore, new-ageism, experientialism, passion, intuition, and inanity persist and may be expanding, if not as systems of belief, then certainly juxtaposed to science. A more virulent criticism is the postmodern claim that science is not truthful or real. From this assumption, the notion of 'scientism' arises: science is powerful and pervasive, but is only one of many ways of understanding (epistemology) the natural and social world; scientific truths and realities, like all others, are socially manufactured.

Certainly, the truth and reality of science and scientific medicine can be questioned. But then so can that of scientism and medicine's 'snake-oil' surrogate (complementary–alternative medicine (CAM).

SCIENTISM

Scientism is a sociological idea that typifies science thus: scientific knowledge is supreme, and the intellectual territory of science is boundless; that is, all natural and social life and events can (eventually) be explained through science. Therefore, science stands above all other epistemological explanations (such as religion, spirituality, metaphysics, and philosophy). Ultimately, only science can (and will) uncover truth and reality. Scientism implies that this typification is fallacious. However, scientism is also based on a fallacy – that of the straw-man.

Lewis Wolpert, Professor of Biology, University College London; Richard Dawkins, Professor of the Public Understanding of Science at Oxford University (2006); Steven Pinker, Johnstone Family Professor of Psychology at Harvard University (2003); and Ben Goldacre (2008a), British-trained medical practitioner and journalist, believe fervently in science. They are the scientific purists that the proponents of scientism are criticising. Dawkins, Wolpert, Pinker, and Goldacre regard science as the only way to understand the natural and social phenomena. Moreover, they are science evangelists. They insist that scientific rules and results should be disseminated vigorously throughout society. They assail what in their view are the abuses of science (for example, the immorality of using scientific discoveries for warfare), and threats to rationalistic thought (the postmodern position that everything and nothing is believable; the absurdity and dangerousness of religion:

I find it ironic that, whenever I lecture publicly, there always seems to be someone who comes forward and says, 'Of course, your science is just a religion like ours. Fundamentally, science just comes down to faith, doesn't it?' Well, science is not religion and it doesn't just come down to faith. Although it has many of religion's virtues, it has none of its vices. Science is based upon verifiable evidence. Religious faith not only lacks evidence, its independence from evidence is its pride and joy, shouted from the rooftops. Why else would Christians wax critical of doubting Thomas? The other apostles are held up to us as exemplars of virtue because faith was enough for them. Doubting Thomas, on the other hand, required evidence. Perhaps he should be the patron saint of scientists.

(Dawkins, 1997)

These scientific purists fear the swamping of society with asinine, uncivilised, and destructive thinking and customs when what is needed are more constructive analyses and answers from science about such social problems as poverty, global warming, and disease.

The history of science is not one of simple progression. To begin with, science did not and still does not evolve through positive linear forward movement towards greater understanding. Science stutters along, backtracks, jumps forward haphazardly, plausibly, serendipitously, as well as in great leaps, at times surpasses, overtakes, or accompanies myth (Gribbin, 2003).

The ancient Greeks set in place the propositions that were to become modern Western science, having learned from the ideas of previous civilisations (for example, Babylonian and Egyptian). The embryonic science of ancient Greece covered medicine, astronomy, cosmology, geometry, mathematics, electricity, magnetism, human biology, zoology, and geography. What the Romans did for science was to add engineering and technology to the knowledge of the Greeks, and extend medical knowledge. Of course, the science of the Greeks and the Romans coexisted with myth (Lindberg, 1992).

In the European Dark Ages and Middle Ages, while myth ascended (especially that of religion), it did not fully displace Greek and Roman science, and Islamic, Indian, and Chinese science also survived. For example, Nicolaus Copernicus (1473–1543), calculated the positions of the planets and pronounced that earth revolved around the sun. Galilei Galileo (1564–1642) calculated that objects with unlike mass will fall at the same rate, and designed an effective telescope.

Science began to reassert itself in the seventeenth century with the beginning of the European Enlightenment philosophical movement. By the eighteenth century, political liberalism and epistemological rationalism heralded the 'Age of Reason'. Voltaire (1694–1778) campaigned against injustice, intolerance and bigotry, and for science. René Descartes (1596–1650) generated ideas that led to the foundation of modern philosophy and mathematics (Descartes, 2007; orig. 1637). Sir Isaac Newton (1642–1727) formulated laws of gravitational force, calculus, optics, and motion and, along with the sociologist Auguste Comte (1798–1857), the deductive method of testing hypotheses – a version of science ('positivism') adopted by most of today's Western-inspired scientific community.

Gerard Delanty (1997) has catalogued the core tenets of positivistic science:

(a) scientism – only scientific knowledge is credible;
(b) empiricism – we only know what can be observed, and the experiment is the basis of scientific observation as it can reveal cause and effect relationships;
(c) all knowledge is susceptible to the techniques of natural science;
(d) there is a reality that can be studied, and science stands objectively and value-free outside of this reality;
(e) internally coherent and universal laws exist and cross over bodies of knowledge.

Industrialisation in the eighteenth century provided the opportunities to apply the ideas of the Enlightenment innovatively and expansively. Industrialisation and scientifically informed technology were inexorably interlinked with capitalist expansionism, and that expansionism in the twenty-first century has gone global.

Science (and technology) are the backdrop to everyday human performance in the twenty-first century. Virtually all of the activities that humans engage in, or aspire to, have a technical basis that comes from science. However, despite its cultural voracity, much of the public seem not to understand much about science. The dangers to the ideals of the Enlightenment from old and new anti-science movements are examined in the journal *Public Understanding of Science* (Einsiedel, 2008). The journal registers the persistent misinterpretation of scientific endeavour by, and scientific illiteracy of, the public (for example, concerning human cloning, biotechnology, and paediatric vaccinations).

Scientific purists consider the attitude of the public towards their preferred doctrine, as one of educational or intellectual deficit. Sociologists of science tend to consider scientific purists as ill-informed or intellectually elitist about the public. Apart from postmodernist rejection of science as a superior version of reality, an interactionist perspective posits that it is disrespectful not to recognise the value of the meanings people attach to their (techno-scientific) reality.

Apart from these external criticisms, scientific purism is also susceptible to 'in-house' censure. Some 'impure' scientists acknowledge that they haven't got, and may never have, the answers to everything. Moreover, they accept that scientific 'fact' springs from theories and that many if not all of these theories (even the most hallowed) will be modified and some may be dumped. That is, scientific knowledge is concerned with objectivity but is also speculative and transformative, and succumbs to social influences in its production. Many important theories in science remain unverifiable (big bang, dark matter, superstring-M theory, and most if not all aspects of evolutionary psychology), and may only become verifiable if funding, public and political interest, and opportunity collide. That does not mean, however, that scientific knowledge is fabricated as the postmodernist has it, merely that it has a convoluted developmental trajectory.

What became known as the 'Kuhn and Popper Debate' took place in the 1960s and highlighted a central and continual in-house disagreement about the nature of science. On the one side was Sir Karl Popper, a philosopher of science, who argued for a particular version of scientific purism. On the other side was science historian Thomas Kuhn who, while not antagonistic to science, reasoned that science was far from 'pure' because it was affected considerably by society (as well as the psychology of scientists).

For Popper (1959), science is not about establishing constant truths – in his view an impossible objective. Science should proceed by attempting to falsify correlations between events or phenomena (variables). Just because a stone falls to earth from a tower or an apple from a tree at a specific and measurable rate of acceleration, and does so thousands of times, this does not guarantee it will happen the next time. The belief that all swans are white, with or without the back-up of empirical research, however, is not a scientific conclusion as it doesn't allow for the possibility of one black swan being discovered. Hypotheses (the testing of the relationship between variables), posited Popper, should be formulated in such a way as to be receptive to being proven wrong. If they cannot be proven wrong, then this is not science, he argued. A correlation between the Freudian 'id' and an individual's violent performance is not open to falsification because, although violence has a reality, the id exists only in the abstract (and therefore such tests are of no interest to the scientist). A correlation between smoking cigarettes and lung cancer can be falsified, and therefore falls under the province of science. That is, it is logically feasible to reach the conclusion that there is no correlation between smoking and cancer (and a 'null hypothesis' based on testing a non-correlation becomes one way of enacting the principle of falsification).

However, this view of scientific advancement as an unremitting journey towards truth (or at the very least travelling away from falsehoods) was challenged by Kuhn (1962). Kuhn argued that there are long periods of 'normal science' during which researchers merely accepted the presumptions of their predecessors. Scientists in these periods operate within an accepted paradigm, and for the most part do nothing more than address particular puzzles that are internal to that paradigm. Only those problems are researched, and conclusions sanctioned, that are 'plausible' to the paradigm. Any evidence that springs up during the 'normal science' period seeming to contradict the precepts of the paradigm are dispensed with through ridicule or are contained by the setting up of theories that are in tune with the paradigm. The scientific community, therefore, was 'normally' self-indoctrinating and self-perpetuating. However, argued Kuhn, at various times in the history of science, the build-up of evidence repudiating the accepted paradigm becomes so great that its tenets and methods start to lose their legitimacy. At this point an era of 'revolutionary science' begins, and the 'normal' scientific hegemony disintegrates. Revolutionary periods are times of turmoil in science, with much uncertainty and contention. Eventually, however, the revolution abates, and a new paradigm emerges. Then a period of 'normal science' based on this new paradigm begins – until the next revolution. The new paradigm, however, while different, is not necessarily an improvement on previous paradigms.

Adopting a Khunian perspective, it could be argued that normal (scientific) medicine is being displaced by revolutionary (complementary–alternative) medicine. Just as scientific medicine had banished myth-medicine to the epistemological graveyard by the twentieth century (at least in the West), so in the twenty-first century it is itself under threat of epistemological burial.

However, as with all political, economic, military elitist regimes scientists (certainly those of the purist bent) continue to extol their own worthiness and the unworthiness of proto-revolutionaries. Indeed, 'epistemological arrogance' is at the heart of what Nassim Taleb (2006) argues is the delusion of normal science today. Taleb, in his book tellingly titled *The Black Swan*, argues that science can only convince itself and try to convince everyone else that the universe and its contents can be understood by controlling what can be accepted as robust knowledge. For Taleb, science is intellectually fraudulent. Science appears to proffer truth, understand reality, and provide accurate predictions, but this is only because science has set out its own rules and concepts. Taleb argues that the natural and the social world are much more prone to random happenings (and the occurrence of 'Black Swan' intellectual googlies) than science allows itself and its audiences to acknowledge.

The reality of normal science, however, does not fit the model presented by either the purists or their detractors. Science is not a homogenous discipline with a rampant hegemonic praxis, nor has it united through one methodology (falsification or otherwise). If science is a community, then it is a very fractious one with vicious internal feuds, subdivisions, and continuing procedural and epistemological disagreements (Fuller, 2007a; 2007b).

Steven Rose (1997), Professor of Biology at the Open University, illustrates this point well. He uses the allegory of five biologists enjoying a picnic by a lake when a frog jumps out of the water. This causes a discussion among them about how and why the frog can jump. Each biologist has a particular theory, all of which have been verified by extensive empirical observation.

First, the physiologist argues that the frog jumps as a direct consequence of the muscles in its legs contracting. These muscles are able to do so because of signals in the motor nerves of the frog's brain, which have originated from images of a nearby snake hitting the frog's retina. The second biologist, an ethologist, states that the physiologist has only explained *how* the snake jumped and not why. The frog has learned the behaviour of jumping away from predatory snakes in order not to be eaten (perhaps as a result of its own near encounters, or from seeing other frogs being caught in this way). The third biologist, who studies development, suggests that the frog can jump because through its stages of growth (fertilised egg, tadpole, to mature frog) its nervous system has been 'wired up' in such a manner as to make jumping in these circumstances automatic. Stepping into the debate, the fourth biologist, an evolutionist, claims that the frog jumps when in the vicinity of snakes because an evolutionary message, tied to its genetic make-up, has been passed down from its ancestors. Finally, the fifth picnicker, a molecular biologist, pronounces that all of the other explanations are wrong. To understand jumping frogs, we have to examine the minute details of the chemical properties of muscles and nerves, as this is where the biological events that mould such behaviours as jumping take place.

Furthermore, the social contamination of science is undeniable. What is studied, how it is studied, and how results are disseminated depends in the main on finding funding. Finding the funds to carry out research depends on the interests of the funding provider. Politicians are more likely to fund research that fits with their policies. Tobacco companies, breweries, and arms manufacturers understandably are unlikely to fund projects that aim to investigate the damage that smoking, alcohol, and guns do to health. If an organisation does provide funds, it may well 'manage' the results to further its own interests. Fighting as ever for purity of science (specifically, for the tightening of the rules over how research is conducted and results disseminated), Goldacre records the manipulative habits of the pharmaceutical companies following the extensive coverage in the media that the widely used and highly profitable antidepressant Prozac may be no better at improving mood than a placebo:

[D]rug companies have repeatedly been shown to bury unflattering data. Sometimes they bury data that shows drugs to be actively harmful ... But there are also more subtle issues at stake in the burying of results showing minimal efficacy ... The pharmaceutical industry is very imaginative ... For instance, sometimes companies will publish flattering data two or three times over, in slightly different forms, as if it came from different studies, to make it look as if there are a lot of different positive findings out there ... Worse than that, companies often move the goalposts and change the design of a trial after the results are in, to try to massage the findings. This is just a taste of the tricks of their trade ...

(Goldacre, 2008b)

The imaginative manipulation of medical research by pharmaceutical companies includes the 'ghost-writing' of research papers and paying prestigious medical academics and practitioners to appear as authors (Fugh-Berman, 2005). Needless-to-say, such papers have a tendency to promote the products of the relevant company.

However, following the rules of normal science may be equally as manipulative, although the mendacity of normal scientists is not of the same order as that of the corporate drug barons. A key rule of normal science, including medicine and the other disease disciplines, is 'peer review'. Sense about Science (2008), the science lobby group, hallows peer review as the most objective way of assessing the value of research, thereby allowing publication of the findings in 'peer-reviewed' journals. The selection of reviewers, however, is a prejudiced process – made by editors or recommended by other reviewers. Moreover, the selected and selectors are already part of normal science. Far from being objective, peer review is a pooling of subjectivity.

Furthermore, science cannot avoid the contamination of morality. Whether it is atomic weaponry, abortion, hybrid human–animal embryos, 'saviour twins', or pan-industrialisation, science is caught in a myriad of moral dilemmas. A refusal to opine on morality does not negate or delegate the moral/immoral consequence of scientific research. Ignorance of the law or absence of intention will still attract a guilty verdict in the courts. Similarly, scientists are morally liable for what they probe and concoct.

Simon Blackburn (2006), Professor of Philosophy at Cambridge University, argues that the search by scientists for truth and reality is a worthwhile pursuit. However, scepticism should be adopted about whether this goal will ever be achieved, no matter how laudable. For Brian Goodwin (2007), Professor of Biology at the Open University, scientific knowledge can only be an interpretation of reality. Subjective opinions and social processes inevitably interfere with the search for facts. Goodwin's solution is the formation of a new culturally sensitive and holistic science, which understands these interferences. Blackburn and Goodwin are, as is Helman, de facto sociological realists.

The realist's approach offers a rectified account of what the scientific endeavour is capable of, without needing to follow the 'nothing is real' mantra of postmodernism. As Dawkins, presumably with a postmodernist air-travelling-conference-attendee in mind, so deftly states:

> When you take a 747 to an international convention of Sociologists . . . the reason you arrive in one piece is that a lot of western-trained scientists and engineers got their sums right. If it gives you satisfaction to say that the theory of aerodynamics is a social construct that is your privilege, but why then do you entrust your air-travel plans to a Boeing rather than a magic carpet?
>
> (Dawkins, 1994)

What Dawkins does not appear to appreciate is that aeroplanes, while clearly scientifically technological, do have contending cultural overtones. They have at various times been construed as exemplifying the ingenuity of industrialised society, dramatic cinematic settings, environmental cataclysms, and deified symbols of pre-industrialised cargo cults.

However, the invention of aeroplanes is not as scientifically unsound as medical intervention. Aeroplanes do fly, but a significant proportion of medical diagnoses and treatment are ineffective. Realism provides an insight into why so much of medical advice based on 'evidence' seems either to be contradicted by advice from other 'evidence', or is at odds with human intuition and experience. That is, the science of medicine has evolved a fair distance from mythology but not nearly as far as modern aviation has from gliding. While aeroplanes can excite passion, artistry, and religion, humans are passionate, artistic, and religious.

MEDICINE

The long association of science (and technology) with (Western) medicine has shifted from being an ally to being fully incorporated into its modus operandi. That is, medicine is no longer just relying on science and its technological outpourings, but *is* science and vice versa. The art of doctoring has been replaced by what medical practitioner and anthropologist Cecil Helman calls 'techo-doctoring' (Helman, 2006).

The prestigious American Association for the Advancement of Science (AAAS) claims to be the leading voice for scientists internationally, with the aim of advancing the take-up of scientific knowledge generally in global society. Since 1880 it has published the prestigious scientific magazine *Science* in order to help achieve that aim. *Science* has a readership of one million. Around 3,200 articles, directly relating to medicine have been published in *Science* during the years 1995–2008 (AAAS-*Science*, 2008).

The other disciplines of disease are heading in the same direction. However, for some (especially nursing), it is not pure science that is being occupationally internalised, but a mixture of 'hard' (quantitative) and 'soft' (qualitative). 'Soft' science is a defilement of the purity of the positivist empirical-deductive method based on the testing of hypotheses derived from theory, and is more akin to interactionist sociological method and Helman's rapidly disappearing 'art' of medicine.

Internationally, the hierarchical ranking of evidence continues to place results derived from 'hard' scientific method such as randomised-control trials (RCTs) as superior compared to those from 'soft' scientific method such as interviews. The choice of scientific method is both a cause and a consequence of status differentials for the disciples of disease.

Medicine is adept at proclaiming both its scientific embroilment and the merits of its scientific evidence. The media regularly report on present and potential medical successes and employ specialist journals to exult over scientific medicine. For example, Alok Jha, science correspondent of the British newspaper *The Guardian*, writes exuberantly about the prospect of science and medicine curing a gamut of disease:

> Scientists have made a major leap in unravelling the genetic causes of seven common diseases, including diabetes, arthritis, and high blood pressure, by completing the largest analysis of the human genome. The discoveries pave the way for improved treatments and possible cures for the millions of people in the UK who develop the diseases every year.
>
> (Jha, 2007)

> A pioneering technique that uses the body's nerves to bypass spinal injuries could help thousands of people to regain feeling, and possibly even the use of paralysed limbs, scientists say. Using similar principles to heart bypass surgery, where veins from a patient's leg are used to get around an artery blockage, scientists in the US have shown that nerves can be used to circumvent spinal damage and reconnect the brain to the body.
>
> (Jha, 2008)

Paradoxically, the media is also very fond of exposing the calamities and culpabilities of doctors (and the odd incompetent nurse or midwife). Occasionally, a medical murderer hits the news (and the odd serial-killing doctor), and such a story can run for years. However, the reason medical murders become notorious is largely because they are so rare (or rather the perpetrators are rarely caught). What is much more frequently presented, giving a negative impression of doctoring, are blunders, some of which result in loss of life but through negligence rather than malevolence, as these two reports from British newspapers (*Evening Standard* and *Daily Mail* respectively) demonstrate:

Blunders by doctors [*sic*] killed runner
A young film assistant died from testicular cancer after doctors failed to diagnose his condition for a month. Matt Elmy went to his GP as soon as he realised something was wrong, but was told

it was probably an infection. He was diagnosed only after going to hospital in agony and refusing to leave. By then cancer had spread to his brain, lungs, liver and lymph system.

(Hopkirk, 2005)

Hospital blunders 'kill 34,000 a year'
Medical blunders kill an estimated 34,000 patients a year, according to an official report.

(Tozer, 2005)

Goldacre, in his publications and on his website, sets about those who abuse, misuse, or omit science, particularly when they have the temerity to interfere with the scientific purity of his own profession of medicine. He becomes particularly exercised over what he considers are the outlandish assertions of some CAM therapists (notably, nutritionalists and homeopaths). Goldacre's (2008c) anger and ridicule was in full flow when he reacted to a widely reported medical 'miracle' about the re-growing of a man's missing finger. The finger (or a large part of it) had been sliced off accidentally. 'Pixie-dust' made from pig-extract, so the story ran, sprinkled on the stump caused a fully working new digit to arise.

Goldacre appeared on and wrote in the media explaining (passionately) the basic failure of journalists to appreciate that there was no 'missing finger' in the first place. According to Goldacre, having studied pictures of the said finger which were shown in the media, only tissue around the distal phalanx was missing. Second, such missing tissue would normally re-grow without help from 'pixie-dust'. Third, the journalists delivering the reports, suggested Goldacre, did not seem to understand how clinical investigations work (that is, through randomised and controlled trials), and therefore were unable to separate good science from bad science. Therefore, they confused daft stories such as this one from those that have robust evidence to support their implications.

For Goldacre, scientific medicine is not only important (because it shows truths about disease) but also is elegant and beautiful (that is, it encloses and exudes passion and artistry). His mission seems to convince everyone else of its concrete and aesthetic merit.

However, while medicine is undoubtedly life-enhancing, exquisiteness is somewhat tarnished by its schisms. As with science, there are very different forms of knowledge and treatments within and across the various medical specialisms. Little common practice exists between geriatricians, paediatricians, and orthopaedic surgeons, and each of these has its own internal subdivisions. The profession of psychiatry encompasses not only drugs, electricity, and surgery, but also 'talk'. The latter can be underscored by humanistic, cognitive-behavioural, or psychoanalytical theory, which themselves are disunited perspectives.

However, all of medicine's schisms, in principle (if not in practice), assign scientific measurement and verification as the ideal. Moreover, revolutionary advances in physics, chemistry, mathematics, computer technology, molecular and cell biology, and pharmacology have been devoured by medicine. The scientific mapping of the human genome is anticipated by medicine to forestall or find cures for hundreds of diseases.

However, the medical profession, even with the aid of a flourishing science, has still not actually conquered heart attacks, many cancers, strokes, AIDS, or even the common cold. Despite improvements in treatment, the number of diabetes and asthma sufferers continues to grow; antibiotics are beginning to be considered a scourge because they reduce the resistance of the population as a whole to disease; and pulmonary tuberculosis, malaria, and cholera remain endemic in many parts of the world. While psychiatrists avow great achievements in tackling mental disorders, at best they are only alleviating symptoms. The health of the poor in the industrialised world, while improved overall, has become worse relative to that of the rich, as has the health of the majority in developing countries compared to that of Western populations.

Furthermore, it is open to debate just how robust science applied to disease is, and how much 'evidence-based-practice' there is actually being employed by doctors, nurses, midwives, and the rest of the disease practitioners. Professor Richard Smith, editor of the *British Medical Journal*, acknowledges the poor scientific quality of medical knowledge (Boseley, 1998). He states that less than 5 per cent of articles from the 20,000 published medical journals worldwide are scientifically rigorous. The results of studies reported in these journals were often contradictory, biased, and shouldn't be generalised although they often are, and some may also be fraudulent.

Also, 'evidence' is mediated through interpersonal communication processes between patients and doctors or other practitioners, and the specific social circumstances of the patient (Haynes *et al.*, 2002). In any one situation the patient's clinical state and circumstances may predominate. For example, a patient suffering chest pain while climbing a mountain might have only an aspirin and hope as treatment. But if he/she had chest pain and full health insurance while within the vicinity of a fully equipped private hospital then he/she would probably be surrounded quickly by half a dozen 'machines-that-go-ping' (Monty Python, 1983). A patient's beliefs (for example, about blood tranfusions, or the sanctity of life, or the acceptance of death) may modify or completely reject 'evidence'. Taking Goffman's dramaturgical view, 'evidence' is not making the decisions about medical care but rather it becomes part of scene-setting in the drama of negotiating decisions.

Crucially, the evidence-based movement is vulnerable to criticism for its reliance on the RCT as the gold standard of research methodology. RCTs involve supplying one group of people with a drug, surgical treatment, or psychotherapy. Another group is given a placebo. Neither group is aware of whether they are receiving real or spurious medical intervention. Responses from both groups are compared, and possibly these are then compared with a 'control group' which has received no interventions at all. However, most trials conducted in this way have small samples, are confined to particular groups of people (for example, patients in one or two hospitals, or self-selecting volunteers), or are stopped early so that the commercial possibilities of treatments can be realised (Trottall *et al.*, 2008).

Therefore, it is exceptional to be able to make generalisations to the whole of the population unless trials have been conducted repeatedly over a long period of time and in conjunction with other methods such as epidemiological studies. However, generalisations are commonly made from these sorts of research studies.

Moreover, RCTs are based on a fundamentally defective statistical formula. Robert Mathews (1998) demonstrates that 'tests of significance', the very heart of scientific analysis, are actually based on a subjective assessment of probability. That is, the setting of the dividing line of '0.05 per cent' for evaluating the chance of an outcome being caused by an identified phenomenon was chosen in 1925 by Ronald Aylmer Fisher (who had attempted to correct a fault in a previous statistical theorem formulated by Thomas Bayes) because it was 'convenient'. The consequence of this arbitrary calculation of what is and what isn't significant is to exaggerate the importance of findings and produce false justifications for accepting highly implausible conclusions. This, argues Mathews, is why so many scientific and medical 'breakthroughs' discovered under experimental and/or laboratory conditions do not perform as such when in general circulation, and why there are so many contradictory results from studies examining the same problem. One study tells us not to eat butter, whereas a subsequent one indicates that eating butter will do us no more harm than eating margarine. Another study suggests that drinking red wine is actually healthy, a second study that any type of alcoholic drink is health-enriching, and then a third that all alcohol should be avoided. These research flukes, for Mathews, are the result of the flaws in science.

Hence, conclusions from research trials cannot be held as infallible realities. However, it is somewhat disingenuous to accuse scientists of making such affirmations. The results of testing hypotheses in scientific publications are usually couched in tentative terms. The media, not scientists, announce that red wine, meat, margarine, coffee, or tea, can cure disease, and at some time later inform the public that these products are too dangerous to consume even in moderate amounts. The public, understandably, are not interested in deciphering complex research reports, but take an overall impression from what is being presented. This leads to facile interpretations of research outcomes. Scientists are well used to not declaring causal pathways between, for example, cholesterol and fatty foods, but to speculate on what the 'associations' might be between these substances. The media and the public, however, infrequently discriminate between 'causality' and 'correlation'.

Moreover, medical science, slowly and somewhat reluctantly, is coming to accept more 'soft' scientific evidence, and it is no longer unusual to find qualitative research reported in prestigious medical journals. Furthermore, it is not so unusual to come across 'hard' scientific evidence in the journals of 'soft' disease practice such as nursing.

Nurses are not just 'softer' than medicine. Along with some other disease practitioners (such as occupational therapists) nurses endorse and employ the non-scientific (and at times fervently anti-scientific) techniques and concoctions of complementary–alternative medicine.

Rampant and comprehensive global consumerism (whether considered to be part of capitalist society or postmodernism society) has entered the health/disease arena in a very big way. Whether preventative or curative, CAMs are trendy and lucrative commodities. About 33 per cent of the population in the USA and 65 per cent in Germany (Hirsch, 2002) use CAM. The London-based Diagnostic Clinic (2005) reports from a survey it conducted that the majority of British people believe CAM to be as valid as scientific medicine. In the UK alone there are at least 50,000 CAM practitioners, and globally billions of US dollars are spent on CAM furnished by a multi-billion US$ industry (Tallis, 2004; Wray, 2006).

Charles Windsor is a complementary–alternative medicine zealot. He wants CAM to become part of disease care in Britain, and for CAM and scientific medicine to unite their respective strengths as 'integrated medicine' (also known as integrative medicine). Windsor commissioned a report to investigate how CAMs could be used within the British NHS. The report, led by the economist Christopher Smallwood and aided by the research consultancy FreshMinds, was launched in 2005 (Smallwood, 2005). In the report, how the 'big five' of CAM (osteopathy and chiropractic, acupuncture, homeopathy, and herbalism) could be used in the NHS is explored.

CAM is popular, and receives zealous support from the (possible) future King of England. But is it credible? Having a Royal advocate and placing CAM alongside scientific medicine and describing such an arrangement as integrative medicine cannot disguise fundamental contradictions between the two. The whole point of CAM is that it *is* different from medical science. The former focuses on health and holism, while the latter concentrates on disease and what Foucault (1973) referred to as the medical 'gaze' (that is, an increasingly microscopic regard to body and mind dysfunction). Moreover, CAM is frequently underscored by 'alternative' rather than 'complementary' epistemological rationales to that of scientific medicine. Scientific medicine is dogmatically committed to hard empirical evidence, whereas CAM's commitment to science is flaky. Indeed, Irl Hirsch, Professor of Medicine at the University of Washington, USA, suggests that the difference between CAM and scientific medicine can be summed up by saying that the former does not have to adhere to scientific testing whereas the latter does.

While doctors usually do not admit that intuition and experience remain mainstays of their practice, the 'belief' of CAM practitioners in their commodities and therapies can replicate that of the religious fundamentalist. In a similar way to the Baptist preacher using faith in laying-on-hands to install spiritual healing, so personal acclamation and royal assertion is laid-on to support CAM: 'As Patron of a number of health charities, The Prince of Wales has seen at first hand what a difference integrated healthcare has made for many people suffering from ill health' (Windsor, 2005). Scientific medicine has been regulated in one way or another for hundreds of years, whereas CAM has only faced regulation relatively recently. Although tighter regulation of CAM has occurred or is in the offing in many Western countries, it remains relatively easy to declare oneself a 'healer' and distribute capriciously ointments for the mind and body. However, courses that provide certificates to mete out CAMs are proliferating. The choice is between perhaps one or two days information-giving and years of intensive tuition.

CAM encompasses an amorphous and mounting collection of ailments, therapies, and qualifications, making regulation desirable but difficult. However, what exactly is being referred to under the heading of CAM is not just an issue of defining products and therapies, and credentials. CAM conflates tribal remedies and rituals of the witch doctor or shaman, and medieval religiosity and superstition with that of Eastern and Western traditional and modern healing practices (that is, 'old-age' and 'new age' philosophies, spiritualities, pills, and potions).

What Windsor is advocating is the intertwining of two distinctive and incomparable epistemologies: (a) the reasoning from ancient civilisations of Mesopotamia, Egypt, Greece, and Rome, and the European Renaissance, Enlightenment, and industrial epochs (Porter, 2002); (b) the convictions from a matrix of folklore, hocus-pocus, mysticism, and what investigative journalist John Diamond calls 'snake oil' (Diamond, 2001).

When in 1997 Diamond announced that he had contracted throat and tongue cancer, he was inundated with advice to reject scientific medical treatment and use instead one of many suggested 'miracle cures'. Thousands of people wrote to him arguing that he should reject chemotherapy and try various herbs and nutritional supplements, but Diamond became an arch critic of CAM in his book *Snake Oil*. What galled Diamond the most was the uncritical faith expressed by the letter writers in all things 'natural' and their detestation of what they regarded as 'synthetic' (that is, scientific) medicine. Despite the efforts of scientific medicine, Diamond died in 2001 at the age of 47 years.

Professor of Complementary Medicine at the Peninsula Medical School at the universities of Exeter and Plymouth) Edzard Ernst is the most prominent sceptic of CAM. Ernst's view on CAMs emanates from his commitment to science. He insists that he is not against CAM per se, but wants to submit CAMs to scientific scrutiny. Only the ones that have scientific validity can then be included in the lexicon of what he regards as legitimate medicines. For example, he accepts that some herbal remedies do work in a limited fashion. He admits that there is evidence that St John's wort, acupuncture, and hypnotherapy, can also work. After evaluating more than 4,000 research studies relating to CAM, Ernst and science journalist Simon Singh conclude that the majority are based not on credible data but on incredible myth (Singh and Ernst, 2008).

The process of integrating some CAMs within scientific medicine can be argued to be yet another incidence of the medical profession colonising a challenger's territory, cherry-picking assets and doling out its dirty work (as it has done with nursing). Rather than the triumphal infiltration of CAM into the domain of scientific medicine, the latter is becoming the master of the former. Those that fail scientific testing then can be demonised and banished, thereby reinforcing the credibility of scientific medicine (Morrall, 2008a). This is what appears to be happening to homeopathy.

Ernst is very critical of Windsor's campaign to have CAM integrated with scientific medicine. He is therefore not in favour of the Prince of Wales' Foundation for Integrated Health, which recruits general practitioners who are willing to offer a wide range of herbal and other alternative treatments to their patients. Ernst, like Goldacre, directs the rawest of his scepticism towards homeopathy:

Homeopathic remedies don't work . . . Study after study has shown it is simply the purest form of placebo. You may as well take a glass of water than a homeopathic medicine . . . The incredibly dilute solutions used by homeopaths also make no sense, he added. If it were true, we would have to tear up all our physics and chemistry textbooks.

(Ernst in McKie, 2005)

If homeopathy did work, points out Ernst, all contemporary laws of physics and chemistry would have to be discarded.

Joining in the onslaught against homeopathy is *Sense about Science*. Specifically, it condemns CAM usage for malaria declaring that, although homeopathic remedies are advertised (for example, on CAM Internet sites) as having a role in protection against malaria and other serious tropical diseases, they are completely ineffective.

In 2008 the British 'natural' cosmetics company stopped selling homeopathic supposed remedies for malaria after the Medicines and Healthcare Products Regulatory Agency proclaimed such products as misleading and potentially harmful to public health (BBC News, 2008a). Representatives of the company accepted that there was no scientific evidence to support the selling of the drug, but they believed it had been successful as a malarial prophylactic.

For Ernst, personal testimonies and assertions about homeopathic treatment (and other CAMs) stem from the attention patients receive from therapists and the placebo effect of their snake-oils. Realistically, attention and the placebo effect have little to offer the million children who die each year from malaria.

Raymond Tallis, Professor of Geriatric Medicine, University of Manchester, is another arch sceptic with regard to CAM, and points out that the strength of scientific medicine *is* its scepticism. That is, he argues cogently, CAM does not avail itself to systematic critique in the same way that scientific medicine does. For Tallis, scientific medicine is in a constant state of dissatisfaction and transformation, seeking to find better understandings for disease and more pleasant treatments. On the other hand, far from discontent with its knowledge, CAM, because of its 'traditional' roots, is complacent and stagnant (Tallis, 2004).

For Raymond Tallis, Professor of Geriatric Medicine, University of Manchester, the fashion for alternative medicine by both the public and practitioners (largely based in rich countries) is having a corrupting effect on present medical achievements and on the possible triumph over disease. He, like Diamond, regards CAM as analogous to snake oil:

> Of course there is much apparent evidence: anecdotes, patient testimony, endorsements from satisfied customers – the kind of evidence used by the first huckster who sold his first bottle of snake oil off the back of his ox-cart and the first magician to turn his attention to the lucrative business of peddling cancer cures.
>
> (Tallis, 2004: 128–129)

CAM, points out Tallis, is no competitor of scientific medicine in the fight against such killers as cancer, heart disease, and AIDS. Support for traditional medicine in the West, he suggests, comes from misplaced sentimentality about folk-medicine and obtuse cultural-relativism.

SUMMARY

Taking the lead from medicine, the disciplines of disease have already been accepted or are in the process of accepting scientism. That is, science is looked upon as a way of sanctifying and purifying the routines of, for example, nursing, midwifery, physiotherapy, radiography, and psychotherapy. However, science, and what scientists project as evidence, should not be taken at face value. Science is implanted in a social context and therefore, what is cast as real must be assessed sceptically. Equally, any sociological theory that purports to have deconstructed scientific endeavour by asserting that all realities are socially constructed should undergo sceptical scrutiny.

The credibility of science from a realist stance can be summed up by amending Winston Churchill's famous 1947 dictum about democracy thus: science is the worst way of looking at the world except for all the others that have so far been tried (Morrall, 2008a). Scientific medicine, with all of its faults, is and may continue to be, the best option to handle immediate human suffering caused by disease. Whisky was Churchill's personal snake-oil, and, unlike many CAMs, there is no doubt of its real effects (and how it affects reality).

A realist's assessment of the value of sociology might be to accept that, as academics do not deal face-to-face with disease and doctors (along with the other disease practitioners) do, it should contribute imaginatively rather than deconstructively to the diminution of real human suffering. As David Mechanic (2003), the René Dubos University Professor of Behavioral Sciences and Director of the Institute for Health, Health Care Policy at Rutgers University, USA, proposes, the imagination of sociology should focus on building an applied academic infrastructure to work *with* not *against* scientific medicine. Through such an alliance *social medicine* can be regenerated and globalised. The impact of social and economic conditions on health/disease can thereby be appreciated and acted on.

FURTHER READING

Fuller, S. (1997) *Science*. Buckingham: Open University Press.

MORAL ACTION

Join and partake in organisations/networks that combine sociology and medicine (or other disease discipline) such as the UK Society for Social Medicine and the USA Social Medicine Portal.

POWER

4

DOCTOR HAROLD SHIPMAN MURDERED hundreds of his patients. Shipman trained to be a medical practitioner at the University of Leeds. I work at the University of Leeds. I teach medical students about murder. I am not intentionally teaching them how to murder their patients, but it is a worry that I might be doing so unintentionally. They certainly have the power so to do.

Doctors, nurses (some of whom have also been notable murderers of patients, such as Colin Norris who killed patients in Leeds hospitals), the other disease-care practitioners (among whom there are no notable patient murderers), and patients (who occasionally murder their practitioner) all have and use power in their relationships with one another. The social and professional endowment of authority mediates and controls these relationships. To understand the nature of practitioner–practitioner and practitioner–patient associations, the nature of power has to be understood. Without such an understanding, power differentials between disease practitioners will lie uncontested and patient empowerment remains forsaken.

As to whether or not differences in power between, say, doctors and nurses need to be remedied, or patients should be empowered or less controlled, is also contestable and may not be so forsaken. That is, appreciating how global power is distributed and connected to global disease is, I dare to suggest, far more justified morally than is the effort expended by the leaders of nursing, psychology, occupational therapy, and audiology (and others) chasing the occupational status of medicine, or in attempting to persuade patients make decisions about their diseases rather than the practitioner. This is not to negate the other revolutions that need to continue over liberty, egality, and fraternity within disease care, but it is to argue for prioritising. Fighting over occupational remunerative parity and interdisciplinary respect cannot be compared with combating death and destruction from global disease.

It is, however, worthwhile understanding power in disease care, if only to prevent medical (and nursing) murdering.

SOCIAL POWER

The personal characteristics of individuals, their motives, intelligence, eloquence, and beauty modulate social power. A shiftless, obtuse, incoherent, and unattractive practitioner is likely to have his/her denoted power somewhat undermined by an enthused, astute, erudite, and beautiful patient.

Apart from the personal qualities the participants bring to a clinical encounter, power is mediated by the symbolic interaction between therapist and client. Denis McQuail (2005) has analysed the exploitation of power in interpersonal communication. Monopolising the conversation can have the effect of gaining control and achieving a desired outcome. Where dominance occurs and goes unchallenged, the greater is the influence. A person can ensure that a message is accepted by making it coincide with the beliefs of the other person. The influence of the communicator will also be determined by the content of the message. For example, the influence will be greater if the topic under discussion is about an issue with which the other person has no personal experience. Individuals who are regarded as credible and having high social status (as well as physical allure, linguistic and cerebral dexterity, and passion for their subject) will be in a powerful position to impose their opinions.

French and Raven (1959), and Collins and Raven (1969) have formulated a typology through which the meeting point of personal power and social power can be recognised. They divide personal power into a number of categories using criteria derived from statuses ascribed by society:

(a) Expert power: experts are given a powerful social status for their specialist knowledge and skills; although there has been a demise in deference to experts within many Western societies, medical practitioners, lawyers, university professors, architects, engineers, and computer scientists are examples of groups with considerable expert power; the disciplines of disease other than medicine are attempting through their respective profession-alising projects to attain a high degree of expert power.

(b) Coercive power: direct physical control, sanctioned either by the state or by powerful groups within society is exercised over others; police and prison officers, kidnappers, parents, and psychiatrists and psychiatric nurses, legally or illegally, contain physically criminals, victims, children, and patients; indeed, restraint and seclusion in psychiatric institutions is used not only as a controlling technique, but also as a medically condoned treatment (with or without medication also being forcibly administered).

(c) Reward power: emotional or tangible pay-offs are given to individuals or groups in order to readjust their performance; for example, parents use praise and approval to encourage 'good' behaviour in their children; managers of disease services may be given financial incentives when they keep expenditure within preset limits (although curiously and counterproductively services may receive extra financial help when budgets go into deficit); emotional and tangible disbursements are offered to alter conduct by nurses caring for people with learning dis-abilities (mental handicap) to encourage the learning of a new skill.

(d) Legitimate power: formal authorisation is granted by the state or other social institutions to influence and coerce; legitimacy is conveyed through statute and training; law enforcers are awarded legal authority via police academies and bar 'bouncers' are given legal authority through a system of licensing; school teachers qualify to teach but also to act *in loco parentis*; lawyers, doctors, nurses, psychologists, and in some countries psycho-therapists have to be registered with legalised professional bodies before they can practise; doctors and nurses may, through the courts, be given legal authority to force-feed a patient, or to let a patient die.

(e) Referent power: the skills a person may have may be acclaimed (athletes, footballers, musicians, sculptors, surgeons), his/her social achievements (Jesus, Muhammad, Mother Teresa, Nelson Mandela, Prime Minster Winston Churchill, and President J. F. Kennedy) respected, or his/her academic prowess (Charles Darwin, Albert Einstein, Stephen Hawking) admired; where another person has attributes that we wish we had ourselves (for example, a student nurse may try to emulate the qualities of a caring ward sister, or a medical student those of an eminent surgeon), we may become sycophantically infatuated with that person.

(f) Informational power: the accumulation of knowledge has long been regarded as bestowing power; Sir Francis Bacon's dictum (1985; orig. 1597) 'For also knowledge itself is power' in the information age of the twenty-first century is apposite; there are now vast stores of readily available knowledge both in literature and on the Internet. However, the assumption that there has been a general empowerment of the global citizen is questionable; first, empowerment depends on access to these resources and the social capital to filter and apply the knowledge once it has been obtained; second, those who provide the information may well have vested interests (commercial, political, and moral) in how it is presented; third, specific examples of projected shifts in power through access to information, such as an increase in patient-empowerment, underplay the might and dexterity of professional power.

Moving beyond locating power within the individual, his/her symbolic interactions with, and the border at which individuals and society meet are two discordant sociological perspectives. The first considers power to be dispersed throughout society, the second to be concentrated within one or a few sections of society.

For Michel Foucault (1980) power pervades all areas of social life, and alters its site and potency over time. Social power for Foucault is akin to blood flow in the human body, where blood floods the heart houses, but then flows into the cells via large and small interconnected vessels. In society, pools of power accumulate in the heart of government and commerce, but then leak to individuals and collectivities, institutions, and agencies.

According to Foucault, power is therefore diffused and faction-alised as well as imposed and grabbed. Therefore, power is not simply secured by the politically and economically privileged, dictators, and generals, but 'enjoyed' by a variety of social groups and people. Harold Shipman did not derive any financial gain from his killings (his inept attempt at forging his last victim's will resulted in his arrest and eventual conviction). Nor do his killings appear to have been carried out for sexual release. However, he must in some way or another have enjoyed (in the Foucauldian sense) his power to kill.

The profession of medicine (along with other fully fledged professions such as law) has been given powers by the state, and has purposefully striven to expand its power. This it has done for selfless and selfish reasons. That is, the possession and wielding of power by doctors may benefit society, but it also benefits the doctors.

Foucault modifies Bacon's premise that knowledge is power, and argues that certain privileged groups in society (for example, medicine and law) have manufactured their own knowledge in order to authenticate and augment their power. What these groups then imply powerfully is that *their* knowledge is 'truth'. Dispersing this truth across society's institutions reinforces the prestige of its purveyors. The 'discourse' of truth (its knowledge, language, gestures, administrative processes, and technical apparatus) furnishes a regenerative circle of truthful power.

Doctors employ Latin, neologisms, acronyms, and metaphors to describe disease in ways that usually only they comprehend. Their use of waiting rooms, white coats, receptionists, stethoscopes, sphygmomanometers, tests, and scans reinforce further their power. Delegation to nurses and referral to other types of practitioner strengthen their authority.

Counterintuitively, the creation and maintenance of a powerful discourse requires the creation and maintenance of the discourse's subject. The legal discourse requires crime (and the fear of crime) to appear real so that the profession of law can be made real and powerful. The medical discourse needs disease to be reified in order for the profession of medicine to become a powerful reality.

Furthermore, those disciplines hanging onto the epistemological coat-tails of medicine also have a vested interest in making disease seem real. Therefore, these 'paramedical' occupations are reliant on the power of the medical discourse and the power of the medical profession for their power. They are 'para' medical because their power is derived from and relative to that of the profession of medicine. For example, nurse leaders have tried to decouple nursing from medicine and promulgate a mixed-up mantra of health and holism, thereby theoretically diverging from the gaze of medicine which concentrates largely on disease and micro-investigation. However, nursing practice overall remains subsumed by the medical discourse. The power of nursing is dependent upon but is below that of medicine, as is that of most of the other disciplines of disease. Without medicine, the practice of nursing would be largely palliative, futile, and unskilled, or disappear. Hence, any occupational strategy employed by nursing or any of the other disciplines of disease to establish authority akin to or even over that of medicine (as clinical psychology has made attempts to do) is ultimately counterproductive.

However, the medical discourse is a reflection of wider discourses. Asking patients about their exercise, smoking, drinking, and sexual habits, and encouraging them to take more responsibility for preventing their own diseases is connected to historical, political, and economic agendas. The individualism of the Enlightenment, the investment of governments and private enterprise in disease care, the spread of international tourism, and what Anthony Elliott and Charles Lemert (2005) describe as 'the new individualism' arising from global capitalism and scientism, form the background to the medical discourse. Specifically, the shift from religion to rationalism, although not linear and perpetually under threat of reversal, has sanctified the body and mind as a singular entity into which medicine can peer. So, medicine as a discourse and profession would not have the characteristics it has or may not have come about at all had these historical, political, and economic agendas not been effective.

The stucturalist argument, however, is that society doesn't merely offer the background to various powerful discourses but determines the content of them and the performance of their targets. Socially produced identities based on economic class, education, gender, and ethnicity have drastic effects on individuals, including practitioners and patients.

For the structuralist, society is not only far more rigidly organised than Foucault or his postmodernist progeny accept, but power plays a pivotal part in how society is organised. How much power people have to influence society and their personal lives will depend on where they are located in the social hierarchy. Generally, doctors are located higher in the social pecking order than their patients or other disease practitioners throughout the world, and can be viewed as indirectly giving support to the ruling class. An exception was during the Soviet regime in Russia when the social status of doctors was deliberately proletarianised, and in 1953 Stalin wanted 'show trials' in a purge of prominent doctors who were accused of plotting against the state (but he died before they took place). Harold Shipman was also an exception in the sense that although he became a professional with power, he was born into a working-class family.

Those who rule society through the wealth they generate, the political or religious hegemony they exercise, and military might (collectively, the elites), produce the norms, mores, and laws that favour themselves. That is, the elites have no interest in altering the status, only in sustaining their power.

A Western way of living based on individualism and capitalism has become either the goal or the achievement of most of the world. Globalisation has altered the composition of the elites, and Marx's division of capitalist society into two classes (the bourgeoisie and the proletariat) requires much modification. The elites have widened beyond that of the wealthy to those who have the power to disseminate particular cultural values, and to intimidate through the threat of military force.

The elite strata in global society now includes: global corporate executives and owners, and shareholders; the heads of world financial institutions (the World Bank, International Monetary Fund); political and military leaders from the wealthiest countries; and the operators of worldwide electronic media and communication networks; the senior members of the United Nations, especially those who are on the Security Council. Moreover, elites from Russia, China, and India have joined the established elites from North America and Europe. The number of US$ billionaires in Russia went beyond 100 in 2008. Russia has the most billionaires in the world after the USA, which has 415 (Forbes, 2008). The average Russian, however, earns approximately US$6,000 annually, and about 40 per cent of the world's population lives on less that US$2 per day (United Nations, 2008). Staggeringly, the income of the world's richest 500 billionaires is more than that of its 416 million poorest inhabitants (Green, 2008).

The proponents of globalisation consider the spread of the 'free-trade' trading system based on Western-style capitalism, and Western liberal-democratic and consumerist freedoms, to be both economically and morally justifiable. It will make everyone better off financially, and thereby improve the quality of life for all (Legrain, 2003). A report by the Commission on Growth and Development (2008), supported by the World Bank, projected that by 2050 4 billion people will live in abject poverty unless countries with stagnating or declining economies allow capitalist free trade.

However, this trading system is anything but free or freeing. It is highly structured. Already it contains protected markets, trade barriers, and economic blocks, and these are becoming more common, and the implementation of social and economic conditions which, when applied to countries such as Russia, breeds billionaires. That is, the structure of global society once it is uncompromisingly capitalist (and of the type of capitalism recommended by the Commission on Growth and Development, which is supported by the World Bank) *may* raise the poverty line for billions (itself a questionable socio-economic forecast), and *will* replicate the power differentials found in such countries as Russia but on a global scale.

Power differentials cause health/disease differentials. Bethan Thomas and Daniel Dorling (2007) map in their 'atlas of social identity' clear divisions in education, employment, wealth, age, and health/disease based on geographical location within one country, Britain. They conclude that from 'cradle to grave' life chances are dictated by where people reside. The length of a person's life will also be affected by whether or not he/she is located in an advantaged or disadvantaged region. However, globalisation is inducing a shift in social divisions, with gender and social class between nations becoming more pronounced than within nations (Perrons, 2004). There are massive international and intranational inequalities in education, employment, wealth, living conditions, health/disease, and lifespan. The powerless subsistence farmer in Sudan is at risk of dying from disease or violence because of decisions made by global oil, food, and arms corporate chief executives (along with those of Sudanese politicians, military and paramilitary leaders). The powerful corporate chief executive from the USA is likely to live a long and healthy life unaffected by any decision made by Sudanese subsistence farmers.

Global corporations are the power-brokers of globalised capitalism. On a global scale, media magnates, chief executives, and major business and finance investors have overtaken the power of politicians and the military. George Monbiot (2007a) argues that global corporations have become so powerful that they now threaten the foundations of democratic government and the earth, and hence the continued survival of humanity. For Monbiot, Western governments are collaborating in their own downfall because they are ceding their power (and therefore the power of the electorate) to these corporations. He accepts the need for globalised trade and a level of industrialisation that sustains that trade, but only if it is policed to ensure that ecological disaster is averted and democracy is regained.

Such unrivalled and unbridled power has led Robert Hare, an expert on psychopaths, to argue that if corporations were people, they would be psychopaths. For Hare, corporations are psychopathic because they have a lack of conscience and remorse about the resultant damage and abuse in their drive for profit. Corporations exploit already impoverished workers wherever in the world they can find them, and operate whenever they can in a part of the world where health and safety, and environmental regulations are lax. Hare also points out that corporate 'social responsibility' programmes are cynical and superficial attempts to convince the public and their customers that they are not psychopaths but compassionate organisations (Hare in Bakan, 2004).

Moreover, the introduction of more and more socially responsible operations alongside corporate commercial activities could be considered an indication of an increased manipulation rather than magnanimity. That is, as capitalism spreads globally, so there is a greater need to disguise its negative by-product.

The example of food is pertinent here because without basic nutrition people become diseased and die. Vandana Shiva, physicist and ecologist, in her 2000 Reith Lecture for the BBC (Shiva, 2000) titled 'Poverty and Globalisation' reported on what she described as an 'epidemic' of suicides among farmers in the Punjab, India. The previously most prosperous agricultural region in India, social disaster has followed ecological disaster. The heavy use of expensive pesticides, due to the trading demands of global capitalism, has not only caused huge debts to mount up among the farming community, but has also wiped out the natural fauna and created vast stretches of waterlogged land. A six-year investigation by Greenpeace (2006) alleged that some of the largest food companies and commodity traders were responsible for encouraging the illegal destruction of the Amazon rainforest. Virgin forest was being cleared for soya crops to be grown which are then used to feed animals slaughtered to feed European fast-food consumers (mention was made of McDonald's 'chicken McNuggets'). By 2008 the system of global food production, marketing, and pricing has become far more volatile, raising the risk of mass starvation among the poorest peoples of the world and the fear of concomitant mass social unrest. Ironically, swapping the ecologically damaging oil production and use for the less ecologically damaging production and use of biofuels has impacted on the availability and cost of the already meagre diet of the world's poor (Oxfam, 2008; Wahlberg, 2008).

Another germane example is that of working and living conditions. Industrialisation and urbanisation in Europe during the nineteenth century wreaked havoc on human health, but through the actions of workers' unions and political parties, by the mid-twentieth century the workplace and housing have become regulated to reduce, if not eliminate, dangers to health. Perhaps there is now over-regulation in business and accommodation in the West. Not so in developing and underdeveloping countries, where working and living conditions replicate those found during European industrial-isation. Shenzhen is China's most successful 'special economic zone', but economic success comes at a price:

SHENZHEN, China: . . . Zhang, a 20-year-old migrant laborer, lost her identity card and was shocked to find that no factory would hire her without a bribe she could not afford. Desperate for money, she ended up working in a grimy, two-room massage parlor in a congested alley here, where she has sex with four or five men a day.

Shenzhen owed its enormous growth to a simple formula of cheap land, eager, compliant labor and lax environmental rules that attracted legions of foreign investors who built export-based manufacturing industries. . . . Today, however, the costs of Shen-zhen's phenomenal success, from environmental peril to social degradation, stare out from every corner. . . . Some, like Zhang, who are drawn to Shenzhen by the promise of $100-a-month sweat-shop salaries end up being trapped here, literally too poor to leave. . . . But others come from far away and are quickly disillusioned by how little they are able to save living in mainland China's most expensive city or quickly tire of the difficult work under often abusive factory bosses and return home.

(French, 2006)

Pre-eminent linguist and social critic Noam Chomsky (2007) comments that it is these countries that are expected to follow the rules of free trade. When they get into debt by doing so (and they inevitably do because the global market is skewed for the benefit of Western (especially USA but also European) elites, then the World Bank and International Monetary Fund force them to close schools and hospitals. This for Chomsky is cultural and economic hegemon-isation of global society, which the USA will protect and advance with military intervention when necessary. That is, control by the global elites for the global elites is enacted through hegemony and militarism.

Far from being compassionate and magnanimous, for Naomi Klein (2007) capitalism run by global corporations thrives on disasters. 'Disaster Capitalism', agues Klein, makes massive profits from hurricanes, terrorism, tsunamis, civil unrest, and wars. When the population is in 'shock' from a disaster, this presents global corporations with market opportunities because the masses are more willing to accept radical free-market reforms. No doubt there is much money to be made from the 2008 food crisis.

SOCIAL CONTROL

The other side to power, whether structured and centralised or dispersed and localised, is control. Professionals such as doctors may not be aligned unequivocally with the elites but they (and their co-collaborating colleagues from the other disciplines of disease) shore up the capitalist system through their association with the functions of the state. At times, however, there is an active and obvious connection between central and local control. For example, psychiatrists and psychiatric nurses have the legal power to prevent a compulsorily detained patient (and under certain conditions, a voluntary patient) from leaving hospital wards, to enforce treatment either within in-patient facilities or in people's homes.

Every form of human society indulges in measures of social supervision. Without order there would be no society:

> It is a truism that all societies, including the most unjust, unequal, disorganized and anomic ones, manifest certain structured patterns of interaction and routine behaviour which we refer to in aggregate as 'social order'. Otherwise we would not call them societies.
>
> (Scheerer and Hess, 1997: 105)

The state and its affiliated institutions of control behaviour place those who aggravate society into one or more of a long list of deviant categories. Legal, political, religious, educational, and medical institutions all assist in the preservation of acceptable admonishing of unacceptable human performance. People are socialised into patterns of acceptable behaviours, thoughts, and emotions. Threats to the social system – especially if serious enough to threaten those who have power – are mollified, incarcerated, or eradicated by the agents and agencies of social control. In global society, because the elites extend beyond the state, these agents and agencies are acting increasingly on behalf of corporate capitalism.

The social foundations of most countries are intrinsically adaptable and durable. Virtually all are embracing the globalising capitalist market without collapsing. The structural fabric of society is only at risk of total disintegration when it faces extraordinary circumstances such as civil war, invasion by a foreign power, economic collapse or ecological collapse, or is taken over by criminal gangs and warlords. Failing or failed states are likely to be occupied by stronger states or eventually re-establish their statehood.

What is much more pervasive and persuasive than categorical coercion is the myriad of everyday informal networks and interaction, perhaps underwritten by political constitutions and social contracts, which lead to compliance. People are socialised into accepting the tenets and vagaries of a social system through fear of condemnation by the 'agencies of social control', but more effectively by the positive and negative messages disseminated by friends, family, peers, and the media.

103

However, Ulrich Beck (1992) argues that 'risk' has become intrinsic to public and business strategies. Within many spheres in society (for example, health/disease, political, employment, and military) 'risk prevention' and 'risk reduction' policies are rife, and there is a plethora of organisations specialising purely in risk. Alongside the culture of risk, there has been a shift in the culture of control.

In the West, since the 1980s, a new social contract of rights and responsibilities has been promulgated to help smooth the progress of globalisation. People are offered greater freedoms to consume, but as a consequence have to be convinced to take on greater responsibility for their communities and themselves.

Nikolas Rose (2000) points out that the 'good citizen' has become one who self-regulates and is then rewarded with further rights. The 'bad citizen' (one who does not self-regulate) is not just punished but demonised. That is, in what I have termed 'post-liberal' society, the 'bad citizen' becomes susceptible to the discourse of risk thinking, risk management, and the technologies of risk assessment and control (Morrall, 2000; 2006b). Defaulting on the responsibilities of the new social contract invites literal or virtual social exclusion. Those targeted for demonisation range from the 'dangerous classes' (paedophiles, criminal recidivists, prostitutes, noisy neighbours, the severely mentally ill, and psychopaths) to the 'pathetic classes' (the fat, indolent, drinkers, smokers, and self-harmers).

For Foucault (1975), human performance is supervised, regulated, punished, and thereby 'disciplined' into ways that are acceptable to the social order. Moral discipline is particularly significant for Foucault.

The way which social power and control is exercised by the disciplines of disease enterprise to control human performance is through the 'sick role'. For the structural functionalist Talcott Parsons (1951), being diseased is not just about how micro-organisms, neoplasms, disability, or physical and psychological trauma affect the body. Disease is regarded by society as a form of deviance and has to be regulated so that society can operate properly. Too much disease would be socially dysfunctional because the economic system would not be serviced, and there would be an unsustainable demand on disease care and welfare services.

The specific way in which the social contract of the sick role functions is through certification. Although self-certification for the initial stage of a period of sickness has become standard practice for employees in many Western industries, medical permission to be away from work for a lengthy period in the main remains mandatory.

For Parsons, there has to be a formula for allowing a certain amount of 'legitimate' sickness. This formula is a 'social contract' between diseased people and the medical profession, which represents the interests of society as a whole. The medical profession is given social power to control access to the sick role.

Furthermore, Parsons, although writing in the middle of the last century and focused on the USA, remains relevant today. The social control function of the profession of medicine through the sick role is applicable to most Western societies and has not diminished but expanded in some. Britain is an example of a country where, because of its advanced welfare provision, the state is demanding more discipline of patients by doctors:

> Minister's cure for 'sicknote culture': A plan to reform the sicknotes used by GPs in England to sign off patients as unfit for work was unveiled yesterday by Alan Johnson, the health secretary. He said the sickness certificate – unchanged for 60 years – gave GPs no opportunity to tell employers how to help staff get back to work and improve their fitness . . . "The evidence shows that, far from being bad for health, work is generally good for people's health. We want to explore what else GPs can do to change our sicknote culture into a wellnote culture." The 'wellnotes' would set out what tasks a worker could be expected to perform. . . . From October, a medical test will assess what individuals can do instead of focusing on what they cannot.
>
> (Carvel, 2008)

When an individual is given permission by a medical practitioner to enter into the sick role, he/she (reclassified as a 'patient') is accorded a collection of social privileges together with a number of social obligations (see Table 1). The patient is given the right to stay away from work, and has exemption from family responsibilities. Moreover, society confers on the patient the right of not being blamed for his/her sickness. His/her duty, however, is to assist in the smooth functioning of society by being motivated to get well.

Medical practitioners also have a set of social privileges and burdens. The profession of medicine is awarded the right to be the paramount agency in controlling access to the sick role, and receives high status and remuneration for doing so. Furthermore, medical practitioners are given social licence to probe the patient's orifices, emotions, and lifestyle. The socially bestowed obligations of the medical profession are: always to have the interests of the patient at heart when delivering treatment; adherence to stringent guidelines for practice, which are formulated by the profession itself; to undergo lengthy and rigorous (scientific) training, which is also formulated by the medical profession; and to act impartially and impersonally.

Other disease disciplines, such as pharmacy, nursing, and psychotherapy, are in some countries either delegated this social task of controlling sickness by either medicine or the state, or it falls to them because of the absence of medical practitioners.

Medicine, therefore, has become an agency of social control, but for Parsons this form of social control benefits the whole of society not (only) the elites. Medical practitioners contribute positively to

Table 1 Being Sick

Rights of the sick person		Rights of the doctor	
1	Exemption from role obligations	1	Controls entry to sick role
2	Exemption from responsibility for illness	2	Granted access to intimate information and examination
		3	Professional autonomy and dominance
Obligations of the sick person		**Obligations of the doctor**	
1	Must be motivated to get well	1	Acts in accordance with the health needs of the patient
2	Seeks help from and cooperates with doctor	2	Follows the rules of professional conduct
		3	Uses a high degree of expertise and knowledge
		4	Remains objective and emotionally detached

Source: After Parsons, 1951.

the smooth running of that society through their beneficent interventions with patients, and as agents of social control. However, if the society in which they operate is engulfed by globalisation (and most already are or are heading that way), then the sick role is de facto advantaging those already powerful.

Parsons did not believe that his model of the sick role could be found in every case of illness, or that medical practitioners and their patients performed consistently in their respective roles. What he presented was an 'ideal type': a model that could be used to try to understand a particular social phenomenon (in this case sickness), without it answering all of the concerns relating to that phenomenon or removing the possibility of alternative understandings.

However, Parsons' model has glaring faults. Many people are not able to take advantage of their rights when sick. Women who are in paid employment and become ill still tend to have to care for their children and hence cannot easily adopt the sick role. Parsons' sick role may be an appropriate way of describing what occurs in acute illness, but when people suffer from chronic illness, it is less likely that their social obligations will be met. For example, depression is being increasingly diagnosed, but it is symptomatic of depression that the sufferer will not be motivated to get well and therefore he/she cannot take up the obligation to be motivated so to do. Moreover, certain diseases are socially stigmatised (for example, AIDS and alcoholism). Here the individual is blamed for contracting the condition. That is, with these conditions the right to be held unaccountable for contracting the illness is not afforded. Medical practitioners also may not always be working directly for the benefit of their patients. Some are 'in it for the money', others are incompetent or abusive, and a few such as Harold Shipman are murderous.

Parsons' conceptualisation of the patient is one of 'passivity'. Other early sociological research into doctor–patient relationships such as that carried out by Thomas Szasz and Marc Hollender (1956) indicated that for much of the time medical consultations were founded on the patient being passive and the doctor being active. However, Szasz and Hollender suggested this was only one of the three possible variations to the doctor–patient relationship, two of which implied that the latter could have a much more vital role than projected by Parsons (see Table 2). To begin with, Szasz and Hollender conceded that in certain health–disease predicaments,

Table 2 Sick Roles

Type of role adopted	Examples
Active–passive (doctor is active, patient is passive)	Patient is unconscious, psychotic, or toxaemic
Guidance–cooperation (doctor guides, patient cooperates)	Acute conditions with known aetiologies, treatments, and prognoses
Mutual participation (doctor and patient negotiate openly)	Chronic conditions with indeterminate aetiologies, treatments, and prognoses

Source: Szasz and Hollender, 1956.

such as during surgery, when a patient is comatosed, has a systemic toxaemia, or is in a state of severe shock, her or his engagement in the treatment process will be unavoidably inert. In these conditions the power of the practitioner is absolute. However, for many complaints (for example, acute respiratory or genito-urinary infections) patients are involved in their treatment to the extent that they 'cooperate' with medical directions. This level of participation becomes balanced, however, with a number of chronic conditions where perhaps the practitioner is more willing to give up some of her or his control to the patient either because medical knowledge about the disease process is imprecise, or the efficacy of treatments is uncertain (as in, for example, AIDS, Alzheimer's disease, chronic anxiety).

No matter what the deficiencies are in Parsons' model, he made a very valuable contribution to the understanding of human performance when sick. Prior to his thesis on the sick role in the 1950s, there was no well-mapped awareness of such an unlikely part of the human predicament (i.e. illness) being a social, as well as a physical and psychological, phenomenon.

PROFESSIONAL POWER

In twenty-first century Western disease-care systems (and increasingly in developing and underdeveloped countries that may be involved with, for example, the empowerment policies of the World Health Organization), emphasis is placed on patient 'activity'. Way back in the dark ages of doctor-dominated discourse (that is, the last century), general practitioner and sociologist David

Armstrong in the 1980s argued that the main reason for the patient's subjective opinion being listened to in the medical encounter was to assist in the medical objective assessment of his/her condition. From Armstrong's (1984) perspective, therefore, patient empowerment is not what it seems. Patients, observes Armstrong, have for hundreds of years been asked to provide details of their conditions and the circumstances in which these were contracted. Using Foucault's (1973) concept of the medical 'gaze', he suggests that from the late eighteenth century, clinical examinations united the search for 'signs' of disease within malfunctioning organs with the invited expression of 'symptoms' that could lead to a more accurate diagnosis. However, for the most part, the worth of signs eclipsed the value attributed to the symptoms. The patient was asked to speak, was listened to, but not heard beyond helping to confirm or repudiate the significance given to physical indications of disorder. Communicating with the patient was a form of interrogation through which the medical perspective, not the patient's, could be instituted.

However, through the influence of psychiatry (and in particular Freud's belief that there was a direct connection between 'inner thoughts' and bodily manifestations of illness), by the mid-twentieth century the 'patient's view' had become an essential element of the clinical examination. What the patient said had now become important for a diagnosis and as a measure of how the patient was coping with or adjusting to their illness. Moreover, the influence of psychiatry continued to affect doctor–patient encounters so that to 'talk' became part of the treatment within both psychological and physical medicine. However, far from liberating the patient from the dominance of medical perceptions of his or her health/disease, the 'patient's view' entered the epistemological territory of the doctor. It became subsumed within the medical discourse, where, arguably, it remains today, expressive and at times volatile, but hardly ever dominating.

The view of social commentators Ivan Illich, Irving Zola, and John McKnight (Illich *et al.*, 1977) of professions including medicine is that they are inherently disabling for both society and individuals. They can therefore never seep out power but only suck it up.

The reality of continued patient disempowerment seems to have been underscored by a report by the disease services watchdog for England, the Healthcare Commission. Despite decades of promoting patient-empowerment, the report concluded that not even those tasked with its implementation believe that patients are that important, let alone the ones making the decisions. In a survey of staff working throughout the British National Health Service conducted in 2007, less than half of the respondents (155,922) considered patients their top priority (Healthcare Commission, 2008).

However, whatever happens when doctors meet patients, most people for most of the time either do nothing about their subjective illness or, especially given the availability of non-prescription treatments and the highly developed market in 'health' commodities, they self-medicate. Furthermore, patients may give the impression of co-operating with medical advice, but they deliberately reject, ignore, or deviate from given guidelines. Alternatively, they may not follow the directives because they did not understand them in the first place.

Significantly, the degree to which a patient becomes active in her or his treatment may be dictated by the type of disease, but the social grouping of the sufferer is perhaps more crucial. Eliot Freidson in the USA during the 1960/70s recognised that a patient's involvement in her or his treatment may be encouraged, and opinion better respected, and more time spent with him/her, if there is a cultural affiliation (for example, if both are white and middle class) between doctor and patient (Freidson, 1970; 1971). With the advent of the Internet and its never-ending library of medical articles and advice, the better educated and computer literate continue to have an advantage in terms of their active participation in the medical encounter.

Freidson's (1970; 1971; 1988; 1994; 2001) work on professional power also continues to resonate today. Although a committed Weberian sociologist, Freidson incorporates a range of theoretical insights from other social theorists. It was Freidson who highlighted that the professions served primarily themselves rather than their patients or society, and their power was used to guarantee privilege.

Genuine professionals (for Freidson these were primarily law and medicine) realised their power through achieving autonomy over set areas of work and domination over everyone else working in the same field (and, of course, their patients).

Specifically, he argued, medicine has gained its autonomy and dominance through the deployment of a range of effective tactics over hundreds of years. These include: beating its early competitors (apothecaries, butchers, lay-midwives, herbalists, priests); political manoeuvrings (aided by the 'cultural affinity' between doctors and those in authority); social closure (redesigning medicine as an exclusive, self-regulated occupation with its own mystifying discourse); and alignment with science (medicine has adopted science as its epistemological guarantor).

The power of medicine has undeniably become diminished since Freidson first proposed this theory of dominance and autonomy. At the macro-level of sociological analysis, a global elite social stratum has formed with enormous power to determine how the world operates economically and culturally. Middle-class professions may service but are not endorsed by the elite. Doctors along with lawyers and accountants have to choose between being employed by corporations or being unemployed. Moreover, health/disease systems in countries previously wholly paid for by the state are moving steadily towards privatisation and therefore corporate not professional control.

However, it is a case of the glass being half-full not half-empty, and certainly not drained. At the micro-level the profession of medicine still maintains much of its high social status and remuneration, autonomy, and dominance despite managerial intrusion, the popularity of non-scientific and lay health/disease care, the increased sphere of authority and practice given to paramedical disciplines, patient empowerment, and bad press from blundering and malevolent medical practitioners. Doctors may err and murder, but they still are far more politically astute and scientifically assured than any other disease discipline.

Doctors are ahead in the game of professional power. Nurses are also involved in a power game not only in trying to become a profession like medicine, but interpersonally with doctors. Stein (1967) examined how nurses play this game to increase the amount of influence they have over clinical decisions and hospital policies. Doctors participate in the game to help resolve predicaments over routines or treatments where they suspect nurses know what appropriate action to take. Stein observes that what always has to be avoided is an apparent challenge to the power relationship between the two groups: 'The cardinal rule in the game is that open disagreement between the players must be avoided at all costs'

(Stein, 1967: 110). Nurses offer advice tentatively and tangentially to doctors. For example, nurses may indicate non-verbally what medical actions they agree or disagree with. They may raise the possibility of an alternative route to be taken over the management of a patient in such a manner as to not appear to have been suggesting anything other than what the doctors themselves would have wanted. Moreover, doctors may elicit recommendations from nurses by oblique invitation. That is, the doctor does not wish to convey to the nurse the idea that the latter's opinion is of value, other than as an appendix to medical judgement.

Deidre Wicks (1999), using data from interviews she conducted with nurses and doctors in Australia, has attested to how gender continues to mediate nurse–doctor relations: ' . . . gender enters into, constructs, negates and shapes a large proportion of what happens and how it happens on a typical hospital ward' (Wicks, 1999: XIV). However, Wicks highlights the complexity of these interchanges, and further elements of game playing. For example, she suggests that nurses are constantly reinforcing and undermining the gender-basis of the relationship with doctors. That is, nurses indulge in passivity at times, but also are mobile in off-setting medical directives when they consider that these are not in the interests of the patients. Resistance to medical imperatives by nurses is particularly common with respect to practices concerning wound treatments, pain relief, and care of the dying. This ambiguity in role performance occurs as a result of a clash between what Wicks describes as 'oppositional discourses'. However, for Wicks it is not the case that these oppositional discourses produce a distinctive dichotomous relationship between nurses and doctors. For example, there is the discourse of medical science, with its concentration on objectified knowledge. This discourse is most prominent today in how doctors conduct their work, but the precepts of science have steadily infiltrated nursing practice. Moreover, there is also within both nursing and medicine a latent 'bedside-healing' discourse, with a far greater focus on the patient as a 'person' and on 'caring' than happens within the scientific discourse.

The doctor–nurse game in the bureaucratic, multidisciplinary-team disease system of twenty-first-century disease services has become far more complex, differs from country to country, and involves far more players than either Stein or Wicks envisaged

(Reeves *et al.*, 2008). But Stein's model, as with Parsons' and Freidson's, has maintained its relevance. Apart from them providing insights into disease care, they also provide the background for comprehending how Harold Shipman had the power to murder.

SUMMARY

Social power infiltrates all social situations and relationships, including health/disease. Power accumulates, however, in certain parts of society. It may be expropriated by the ruling elites, or disseminate to disparate social groupings. Uncontrolled power can pervert society, encouraging the disavowal of human rights, furnishing health/disease inequalities, and allowing murder.

However, the exertion of power by the state and other social institutions is also indispensable for the perpetuation of society, and for the protection of susceptible groups. Without significant restraining mechanisms, society would disintegrate, leaving only anarchy and barbarism. The sick role is one means by which society controls deviancy to aid social constancy *and* vulnerable people (the diseased).

According to Larry Elliot and Dan Atkinson (2008), the world's social hierarchy is being divorced into the super-poor and the super-rich camps. For them such a population bifurcation is destroying the middle class (including the professions) which has made a positive contribution to society. Ironically, it is also destroying the very financial and business systems that allowed the rich to become super-rich. That is, the super-rich are dysfunctional for global society.

So, professionals overall are not as powerful as they once were. However, if the profession of medicine was to lose further power through the process of empowering patients and lost its game with nurses and other disease disciplines, the sick-role part of the social contract may collapse. If Parsons is correct in his assessment of the functionality of the rights–obligations equilibrium for doctor and patient, and the expediency of medical control over sickness for society, what could supplant this arrangement? It is to think the unthinkable to muse that the sick role may be irreplaceable, and that the policy of patient-empowerment may be as counterproductive for society as the destruction of the middle class has been. Is it far too politically impolite to postulate that doctors are and should be members of the better team in the game of professional power and that rather than continuing in futile interdisciplinary competitiveness, the disciplines of disease should engage in the struggle against the real foe – global disease?

FURTHER READING

Freidson, E. (2006) *Professional Dominance: The Social Structure of Medical Care* (new edition). Edison, NJ: Aldine Transaction.

MORAL ACTION

Five thousand five hundred children under the age of five years die every day from diarrhoea. Scientifically formulated sachets of oral hydration salts can save a child's life; they cost £0.3/ US$0.6 each. Decide how many children's lives you wish to save and send the appropriate amount to UNICEF. Lobby your representative occupational organisation to do the same.

MEDICALISATION

5

MEDICALISATION MEANS THE INTRUSION into everyday life of medical interventions. Sociologists frequently invoke the stance of Ivan Illich (1975) who, in his polemic against the profession of medicine (and all other professions), considers that there has been considerable over-stimulation of 'wants' by people in Western countries.

In the main, sociologists are consistently critical of medicalisation, using the term pejoratively. Generally, the criticism arises from the appliance of a constructionist/postmodernist perspective on health/disease and the profession of medicine. The concept of medicalisation has become accepted as having an element of legitimacy by the medical profession. Such acceptance is unusual for any sociological critical idea, and particularly rare for acceptability to stem from the target of the criticism.

In part, the acceptance of the concept of medicalisation as having a degree of legitimacy is because of its palpability. The medicalisation of everyday life in the West, having progressed slowly for centuries, is now rampant. Moreover, medicalisation is rampaging across global and cyber society, and is doing so all the more successfully because it is encompassing former epistemological enemies. The tactic of embracing threats if deriding them is ineffective has previously served the profession of medicine well, and is doing so once again. Traditional, complementary, and alternative health/ disease care are being increasingly scientised and thereby are succumbing to medical governance.

Novel syndromes, maladies, and disorders are discovered (or as the constructionist/postmodernist would have, 'invented') regularly. A huge variety of social and personal phenomena have become administrated by the medical enterprise.

Menstruation is no longer a natural if unwelcome 'curse', but a medical 'condition' to be regulated. Pre-menstrual tension is not a period of unavoidable (and previously unmentionable) hormonal imbalance, but a syndrome to be soothed:

> Menstruation always did have a scurvy reputation, what with blighting crops and souring milk, but it took 20th century science to discover that women could be possessed by evil spirits before their periods had even begun. In 1931, pre-menstrual days were found to be a time of tension and hostility. They deserved a name of their own: PMT [pre-menstrual tension]. In 1953 Dr Katharina Dalton . . . spotted a multitude of new symptoms, and invented something better: Pre-menstrual Syndrome, or PMS. This majestical syndrome embraces clumsiness, amnesia, fatigue, depression, anxiety, mood-swings – 150 different symptoms! It can account for completely different states of mind: lethargic and energetic; lecherous and unresponsive . . . PMS has been accepted as an excuse for shoplifiting, arson and homicide.
>
> (Bennett, 1998)

A big body no longer signifies simply a big appetite or, as in some Asian and African cultures, high social status, but has become a stigmatised disorder in both developed and developing societies, much to the chagrin of 'fat activists'.

The Fat Activist Task Force, a coalition of activists from San Francisco, USA, formed in 1989 to fight what it describes as 'size discrimination'. Its tasks include:

1 Working with the [USA] Federal Trade Commission to help stop diet fraud.
2 Assisting in a successful campaign to add height and weight to the list of characteristics protected against discrimination in San Francisco.

3 Speaking out against a fat toddler being removed from her home.
4 Helping an LAPD Officer who faced career-ending disciplinary
   action over reporting an offensive "No Fat Cops!" poster in a
   captain's office.

(The Fat Activist Task Force, 2008)

Being miserable, experiencing feelings of exhaustion, and not possessing the work ethic is not merely having a particularly despondent and lethargic personality or an understandable and rational response to the strains and expectations of everyday life, but myalgic encephalomyelitis ('chronic fatigue syndrome'). If these traits occur during the winter, they may become attributed to 'seasonal affective disorder' rather than again an understandable and rational response to perhaps a cold and dim climate.

Being drunk and feckless is no longer a lifestyle choice for some individuals and communities but 'alcoholism'. If drunk and feckless only at weekends, then the individual may be tagged a 'binge drinker' and the community described as having a 'binge-drinking culture'. In countries such as Britain, Ireland, Norway, Sweden, Finland, and Australia, and particular sections of society such as the Glaswegian working classes and Geordies (people born around Newcastle-upon-Tyne in England), university students and young men and increasingly young women in general, have gained a reputation of being especially afflicted. However, humans have been drinking alcohol for millennia, and medical models of alcoholism also have a long history:

> In the USA in 1784 Dr Benjamin Rush, a signer of the Declaration of Independence, published his famous tract 'An Enquiry into the Effects of Ardent Spirits Upon the Human Body and Mind With An Account of Prevention and of Remedies for Curing Them', where alcoholism was described as a 'disease of the will'.
>
> (Helman, 2007: 209)

Schoolchildren are not naughty, bad, or simply stupid (the very idea of stupidity is no longer politically acceptable in the educational setting), but have 'attention deficits' or 'hyperactivity'. Idiosyncratic and inefficient writing and reading has shifted from being learning difficulty to being 'dyslexia'. Killing another human, rather than

117

being categorised as homicide, could be classified as 'Munchausen's by Proxy'. Paedophilia is not just criminalised but psychiatricised with a range of psychological and psychopharmacological treatments made available (although perhaps only in the therapeutic environment of a prison). Being caught with others in a war zone and having bombs dropped in your vicinity becomes 'complete mass conflict disorder' rather than just recognised as a group of people scaring each other witless. Cantankerous, ill-tempered men can now claim to have caught 'irritable male syndrome' in mitigation for their otherwise antisocial behaviour.

Deformity is no longer a variation on human physiognomy, but an unacceptable aberration in a world that venerates very specific types of bodies. Body-parts that are absent, extra, have fallen out, are too blemished, too long, too short, too big, too short, too stiff, too wobbly, too taut, or too slack can be replaced, removed, or invigorated.

In an Internet advertisement for the 'Laser Vagina Rejuvenating Institute of Los Angeles' (2008) in the USA, underneath a picture of the two male surgeons who conduct the treatment (both with broad smiles and very white teeth), the promise is made of enhanced sexual gratification by making the vagina smaller and strengthening its walls. The advertisement also includes the result of the institute's survey in which the question was asked 'Do women want to be loose or [sic] relaxed or do women want to be tight?' Apparently, 100 per cent of female respondents said women want to be tight. No surprise there, then, just as the equivalent question for men about penis size is likely to receive equal unanimity, and for which there are similarly smiley-white-teethed surgeons willing to perform the necessary operation.

Medicine in the twenty-first century has entered cyberspace with readily available medical advice and treatments from orthodox, unorthodox, and distinctly dubious Internet sources run by actual and digital doctors or by 'snake-oil sellers'. This is exacerbating medicalisation, oscillating further the doctor–patient relationship, and heightening ethical dilemmas over the sale of human organs (Miah and Rich, 2006; Nettleton, 2004; Morrall, 2008a).

The medical profession is not unaware of the negative by-products from excessive medical interference with everyday life. For example, the journal of the Public Library of Science *Medicine*

(2006) published eleven articles by USA and British medical experts on the subject. However, the authors tended to blame not doctors but the pill-pushing companies. That is, the claim was made in the articles that pharmaceutical corporations were 'disease mongering' by inventing new and possibly sham disorders. The authors accepted that doctors at times did the same, but then again blamed the pharmaceutical corporations for taking commercial advantage of these discoveries by exaggerating their authenticity and then emphasising the need to offer treatment (which, of course, they could supply). Doctors (and by implication nurses and pharmacists) therefore experience the 'hard-sell' from the drug representatives and advertisements placed in medical journals and succumb to these pressures, which results in unnecessary prescribing or over-prescribing.

That drug treatments are part of a capitalist system of maximising profit is in no doubt, and that the corporations who sell (and push) the drugs take advantage and are vulnerable to the ups-and-downs of the financial markets is beyond question:

> Hyperactivity drug goes too slow for Shire. Shire fell sharply again yesterday on continuing concern about the performance of its Vyvanse treatment. At the end of last month the pharmaceuticals group admitted that sales of Vyvanse – its attention deficit hyperactivity disorder drug – were likely to be at the lower end of City forecasts for 2008. Analysts at Credit Suisse said they were tracking the drug's performance in the key US market, and the latest weekly figures were disappointing.
>
> 'Vyvanse has captured a 7.2% market share as of the week ending 25 April, with a rolling four-week market share gain rate of 0.4%,' the bank said. 'The launch is still tracking at the lower end of our expectations and we believe that a substantial pick-up in market share gains will be required before the end of the quarter to prevent further downgrades.' It repeated its underperform rating and 823p price target.
>
> (Fletcher, 2008)

Michael Fitzpatrick (2000), British general practitioner, argues that we live in an age of tyranny from health/disease scares. Supposed risks from disease are being exaggerated, thereby causing high levels of anxiety among patients. Doctors and the public are being bombarded with counterproductive policies from politicians. Patients then demand treatments when they are actually healthy, flooding the general practitioners' surgeries with erroneous or trifling complaints and requesting pointless consultations with specialists and gratuitous investigations. Moreover, doctors are obliged to contact patients for various health/disease checks, again resulting in possible further superfluous consultations and investigations.

So, it would seem from these accounts that it is not the medical profession that is at fault, but corporations, governments, and patients. Although active in the doctor–patient relationship, medical practitioners seem strangely passive in their relationships with salesmen/women and politicians. However, there are, surprisingly, some doctors in positions of influence within the medical profession who do lay the blame for medicalisation at the door of their colleagues. The redoubtable Richard Smith, editor of the *British Medical Journal*, is one of them. Smith (2002) doesn't lay all the blame for the manufacture of 'non-disease' on corporations, governments, or patients. He recommends that all medical students should read Illich's treatise on medicalisation as part of their training to be doctors.

If medical students did so, however, they would then face difficulty dealing with Illich's solution to medicalisation, which would probably not coincide with their career aspirations prior to reading his book. What Illich offers is a 'radical utopian' answer to the disempowering effect of the professions. He predicts an eventual nemesis for the professions:

> Professional cartels are now as brittle as the French clergy in the age of Voltaire; soon, the still inchoate post-professional ethos will reveal the iron cage of their nakedness . . . But unbeknownst to them their credibility fades fast. A post-professional ethos takes shape in the spirit of those who begin to see the emperor's true physiognomy.
>
> (Illich, in Illich *et al.*, 1977: 37)

Illich advocates the de-professionalisation of all professions, together with the de-industrialisation of the developed world's economic base. Industrial society would be replaced by a system of 'intermediate' technology. He argues also for the retention and protection of craftwork. Technological production would be based on the needs of the community, rather than on the over-stimulated 'wants' created by the monolithic and alienating industrial conglomerates – and the professionals.

The problem with the radical utopian approach is that, apart from spontaneous revolution, there is little elucidation on how industrial society is to go through such a transformation. Nor is there qualification of exactly what is meant by 'intermediate' technology, or what mechanisms would be put in place, on the one hand, to prevent unacceptable growth, and on the other, to ensure against technological decline (Richman, 1987). Moreover, since the 1970s (when Illich began his crusade for smaller scale and locally based economies), the economic agenda has altered spectacularly. Although experiments in 'intermediate' and 'appropriate' technology are proliferating, large-scale industrialisation and global capitalism are the norm.

Taking up Illich's polemical recommendation on how to deal with medicalisation, Richard Smith and journalist Ray Moynihan suggest both de-medicalisation and de-professionalisation:

> Perhaps some doctors will now become the pioneers of de-medicalisation. They can hand back power to patients, encourage self care and autonomy, call for better worldwide distribution of simple effective healthcare, resist the categorisation of life's problem as medical, promote the de-professionalisation of primary care, and help decide which complex services should be available.
>
> (Smith and Moynihan, 2002: 860)

The medical profession through medicalisation contributes to its control role in society which sustains the status quo for the benefit of the powerful elites or manages social change in such a way that doesn't dislodge the power of the elites. This it does obviously when 'social deviants' are diagnosed mad and managed through chemicals or incarceration.

Consider the following situations: A woman rides a horse naked through the streets of Denver claiming to be Lady Godiva and after being apprehended by the authorities, is taken to a psychiatric hospital and declared to be suffering a mental illness. A well-known surgeon in a Southwestern city performs a psychosurgical operation on a young man who is prone to violent outbursts . . . Scientists at a New England medical center work on a million-dollar federal research grant to discover a heroin-blocking agent as a 'cure' for heroin addiction. What do these situations have in common? In all instances medical solutions are being sought for a variety of deviant behavior or conditions . . . the medicalization of deviance.

(Conrad and Schneider, 1980: 28)

However, there is also a far more subtle side to social control through medicalisation. Many (if not all) serious illnesses have social and environmental dimensions, but society is not medicated or surgically readjusted. When a doctor treats a patient for bronchitis, heart failure, lung cancer, obesity, or mental disorder, the focus of the intervention is on the individual. It is the *individual* who attends surgery, strips for examination, has his/her blood sent to the laboratory for investigation, and to whom medication is supplied or on whom surgery is performed. Sick society is not offered a cure, never mind prevention for the circumstances that perpetrate disease in humans.

Therefore, medical practice by individuating public issues such as poverty and pollution reinforces the very social system that is the source of much disease. Moreover, the responsibility of the state to change society is diminished, although doctors carry out remedial interventions on individuals. In developing and underdeveloping countries, this issue is of even more relevance than in the developed countries. There is a moral dilemma over whether or not Western-orientated medical aid delivered to poor and polluted countries, especially if not culturally sensitive, diverts attention (as does other forms of aid) from need to address the structural (political and economic) conditions that are the root cause of the poverty and pollution.

IATROGENESIS

For Illich, the medical profession is extremely damaging in itself to both individual and society. It has put both the health of individuals and society in jeopardy as a consequence of doctor-inflicted injuries and loss of self-autonomy. Illich describes these ill effects of medicine as 'iatrogenesis'. Medical intervention, argues Illich, is such a cause of morbidity and mortality that it can be viewed as one of the most rapidly spreading epidemics of modern times.

Illich was writing in the 1970s, and laid much if not all of the blame for iatrogenesis on doctors. Today, it is not just doctors who perpetrate medicalisation and its penalties, but all of the disciplines of disease. Updating Illich's approach, nurses, midwives, physiotherapists, psychologists, audiologists, psychotherapists, *et al.* are to a greater or lesser extent all guilty of iatrogenesis. Furthermore, the harm from medical intervention can be immediate, delayed, short-term, long-term, minimal, major, direct, indirect, localised, or globalised.

Illich considered three forms of iatrogenesis. First, there is *clinical iatrogenesis*. Here, Illich is referring to the most understandable and evident negative consequences of medical intervention. These include the damage done physically and emotionally to patients from the medication they receive or from surgery they undergo, mistakes in their care and treatment, and from infections caught in hospital.

All pharmaceutical products have side effects (generally, the more toxic the medication, the more lethal the by-product), and approximately 5,000 patients in Britain alone are dying per year from adverse reaction to their prescribed drugs (British Medical Association in Boseley, 2006). Known medical errors seriously harm 1.5 million USA citizens annually (Roehr, 2006), and one in ten patients globally (World Health Organization, 2005). Although the powerless are more vulnerable to medical mistakes, the powerful are not invulnerable:

Doctors in Israel have admitted making a mistake in December when they treated the then prime minister, Ariel Sharon, with large doses of blood thinners after a mild stroke . . . . [T]he anticoagulants given after a minor blood clot two weeks earlier might have caused the debilitating haemorrhagic stroke.

(Associated Press, 2006)

123

Unnecessary operations are on the increase because of the stepping-up of medical liability generating a 'better safe than sorry' mentality among practitioners and insurers (termed 'defensive medicine'); a large landfill site could easily be filled to overflow with the debris from gratuitous laparotomies, biopsies, appendectomies, tonsillectomies, adenoidectomies, episiotomies, gastroectomies, mastectomies, hysterectomies, abortions, caesareans, and aesthetic corrections.

The American College of Surgeons state, as one of their professional principles:

> No operation should be performed without suitable justification. It is the surgeon's responsibility to perform a careful evaluation, including consultation with others when appropriate, and to recommend operation only when it is the best method of treatment for the patient's problem.
>
> (American College of Surgeons, 2006)

Such a proclamation is surely stating the obvious. It is akin to government departments of justice pointing out to police officers that they shouldn't commit crimes, or education authorities telling teachers not to condone ignorance.

However, litigation against doctors is so rife in the USA that a pact between the public and the medical profession will emerge. The American College of Surgeons (2006) records that a survey conducted in 2003 by an organisation called The Health Coalition on Liability and Access reveals that the USA public regard litigation as undermining the availability of health/disease care, forcing some doctors to leave their profession.

Florence Nightingale (1820–1910) firmly believed in hygiene, declaring that hospitals should do no harm. Indeed, Nightingale's instigations of hygienic routines during the Crimean War in the middle of the nineteenth century contributed to the process of medicalising hospitals. She assisted in redesigning hospitals as places where doctors could improve their skills, knowledge, and reputations, if only because their patients didn't die in the numbers they previously had because of the terribly unhygienic conditions. Until then, hospitals had tended to be places that did nothing but harm because they were riddled with infection and thus perceived to be gateways to death (Porter, 2002).

The incidence of disease and death arising not from what the patient brings into hospital, but from what he/she catches while in hospital, is increasingly massively. The hospital acquired infection methicillin-resistant *Staphylococcus aureus* (MRSA), clostridium difficile, pseudomonas, and *Acinetobacter baumannii* debilitate and kill hundreds of thousands of patients (civilian and military) in developed, developing, and underdeveloped countries alike. Moreover, resistance to antibiotics used to fight such 'super-bugs' as well as to fight 'ordinary' infectious diseases is rife globally (Health Protection Agency, 2008).

Social iatrogenesis is Illich's second type of medical misfortune, whereby the whole of society becomes dependent on the medical profession. People become addicted not just to medicines but to the medical profession. Moreover, there is a tendency to use doctors to sort out not just our diseases, but also our interpersonal strife, child-rearing practices, sexual inadequacy, unhappiness, and the side effects of our lifestyle choices and overindulgences. The medical discourse thus seeps into the infrastructure and content of human culture: normality becomes refashioned as deviance through medicalisation:

> Social iatrogenesis is at work when healthcare is turned into a standardized item, staple; when all suffering is 'hospitalized' and homes become inhospitable to birth, sickness, and death; when the language in which people could experience their bodies is turned into bureaucratic gobbledegook; or when suffering, mourning, and healing outside the patient role are labelled a form of deviance.
>
> (Illich, 1975: 49)

Such dependence has, for Illich, made the medical profession extremely powerful. Doctors turn into our priests upon whom we confer such holiness that, like religious leaders, the veracity of their wisdom, while possibly privately doubted, will not be publicly disputed.

Third, Illich posits that clinical iatrogenesis and social iatrogenesis lead to such entrenchment of medical authority in all areas of human life that the individual loses his or her ability to make autonomous judgements. This end product of medical intrusion into how we organise our lives Illich describes as cultural iatrogenesis. Cultural iatrogenesis has incapacitated the individual. He/she is unable to make personal decisions about his/her life, or experience pain, suffering, and death as an inescapable part of existence. Hence, humans have become separated from their own humanity, nature, and reality.

> The modern medical enterprise represents an endeavour to do for people what their genetic and cultural heritage formerly equipped them to do for themselves. Medical civilization is planned and organized to kill pain, to eliminate sickness, and to abolish the need for an art of suffering and of dying.
>
> (Illich, 1975: 138)

Illich recognises that the negative consequences of a physician's or surgeon's interventions have always occurred. Doctor-inflicted trauma has been the result of professional callousness, negligence, and incompetence throughout the history of medicine. Indeed, at times such malpractice has been justified by the medical profession as the inevitable repercussion from administering untried treatments which in the long run will benefit humankind. That is, mistakes have to be made as part of the process of learning about what works and what doesn't in medical practice. However, he makes the point that as medical practice discovers more puissant treatments to fight otherwise untreatable diseases, so the sequela becomes all the more sinister. At its most extreme is the example of inhuman experimentation on humans during the Nazi rule in Germany where doctors conducted trials on those who were unable to object to becoming guinea pigs in the plan to create a master race. However, ordinary medical mistakes and manipulations are everyday occurrences.

HEALTHISM

Robert Crawford has identified a social process that extends substantially the medical intrusiveness into our lives. This he describes as 'healthism' (Crawford, 1980). By the 1970s there had been, observed Crawford, an explosion of commercial and politically sponsored interest in exercise, jogging, diets, vitamins, fitness machines, and anti-stress measures. By the 2000s, healthism had gone much further, bringing an aggressive anti-smoking, anti-alcohol, anti-fat, anti-cholesterol, anti-lazy, pro-fitness, pro-slimness, pro-moderation, and pro-happiness ethic.

The promotion of 'autonomy' over one's life and health is in reality the promotion of oppression. The health police, an amalgam of medical practitioners, nurses, disciplines allied to medicine, politicians, and psychotherapists, are patrolling human performance as never before in human history. In the USA, the principal agency for 'protecting the health of all Americans', the Department of Health and Human Services (DHHS), considers swathes of human performance to merit its advice and intercession. Among many other aspects of health/disease, the DHHS lists as within its remit:

- coping
- eating right
- drinking
- sun, air, home, workplace, school
- exercise and fitness
- general wellness and healthy lifestyle
- smoking and tobacco
- traveller's health
- violence, abuse, and neglect.

In a similar way to Illich, Crawford pointed out that normality as well as deviance was being medicalised. Government health departments, the World Health Organization, and the alternative/ complementary bandwagon consider failure to be healthy as a failure of will. Unhealthiness is now a deviance, healthiness is the model for 'good living', and the healthy are 'good citizens' and the diseased are 'bad citizens'.

A day in the life of an erstwhile unreformed and unhealthy citizen consists of: a pre-breakfast cigarette, followed by a fried and high fat meal (eggs, sausages, 'black pudding', white bread, a beverage with full-cream milk and sugar); a drive to his or her place of employment, where a sedentary role is performed; serial decaffeinated coffee consumption and copious smoking while at work; an alcohol-rich lunch, with chips; chocolate and cake during breaktimes; a drive home via the public house for early evening refreshments; at home in the evening 'couch-potato' leisure pursuits with accompanying alcoholic refurbishment and at least one high-calorie feast; and finally, a cigarette and an uncompleted sexual act before total collapse.

A day in the life of a reconstituted health-conscious citizen consists of: pre-breakfast physical exertions, followed by cholesterol reducing organic porridge, and roughage-containing wholemeal bread; a jog to his or her place of employment, which involves passing a myriad of 'fitness' images displayed in shop windows and the magazine racks of newspaper shops; any food consumed at work consists of (diet) soft drinks, decaffeinated herbal tea, and low-calorie biscuits, and vitamin tablets, which are only eaten after participation in the employer's mandatory exercise breaks; an aerobic session at the local gym precedes an evening meal of vegetarian nouvelle cuisine and two small glasses of (red) wine; and finally a soothing sexual encounter, and the reading of an article on self-improvement, prior to a restful night's sleep.

Healthism, from the constructionist/postmodernist viewpoint, is part of the consumer culture, stimulated by the pharmaceutical companies, media, fashion industries, and sports/fitness enterprises. Health is procured as a commodity, and has become yet another facet of what both structuralists and constructionist/postmodernists might agree is 'conspicuous consumption' (Greenhalgh and Wessely, 2004). Just as the SUV/4WD, exotic holidays, fashionable clothes, and expensive jewellery are flaunted as statements of success and exhibitions of excess, so is the gym membership, access to private health/disease services, toned body, and redesigned genitalia.

It is not, however, just health that is being commodified, but the body. Human body parts and reproductive cells are sold on the Internet. Biotechnology companies are attempting to patent segments of the human genetic code. The unravelling of the human genetic code offers the prospect of major medical advances, as well as the potential for colossal profits if the rights to the knowledge of how genes work are commandeered by capitalist enterprises. The blueprint to life itself will then be for sale.

PSYCHO-HEALTHISM

There is also a proliferation of policies, practices, and commodities designed to advance the psychological well-being of the masses:

psycho-healthism (Morrall, 2008b). Tens of thousands of psychiatrists, psychologists, and psychotherapists, deliver hundreds of different treatments and therapies in an expanding global market of personal troubles.

Medicalisation has been rampant, especially in the area of human life that Thomas Szasz (1972) calls 'problems with living'. However, Mary Boyle (2002) argues that psychiatric medicine has perpetuated a 'scientific delusion' with respect to what psychiatry calls mental disorder. From the medical scientific perspective, mental disorders are diseases of the mind rather than of the body, although there is an acceptance that the Cartesian mind–body split is misleading and therefore of psychosomatic interconnection. From the sociological and social historian perspective, the preferred nomenclature for mental disorder or mind disease is madness because the human performances that fall into this category do so not only or even as a result of disease, but due to its social connotations and causes. For Boyle, the psychosocial complexities that make up what we are as humans, the fallibility of psychiatric diagnosis, and the fragility of scientific and medical knowledge combine to 'deconstruct' such mental disorders as schizophrenia.

Michael Stone (1998) observes that there were more psychiatrists in the last half of the twentieth century than in all of the history of the discipline, thereby achieving a thorough psychiatrisation of human thoughts, behaviours, and emotions. Moreover, social values have been altered because the discourse of psychiatric medicine has entered irreversibly into the culture of Western societies.

The discourse of psychiatry has been substantiated initially through the development of psychoanalysis by Freud, and then as a consequence of the application of pharmacology to mental disorder. In the 1930s and 1940s, new physical treatments (for example, psychosurgery and insulin therapy) were introduced, and then in the 1950s the serendipitous discovery of antipsychotic and antidepressant drug treatments reaffirmed the biomedical base for the treatment of madness. Furthermore, psychiatry has had a considerable boost with the undeniably impressive progress made in medical diagnostic technology: computerised axial tomography; magnetic resonance imaging; neuroimaging; photomicrography; positron emission tomography; and single photon emission tomography. Moreover, the third revolution has been revitalised further with a new wave of psychotropic drugs such as the selective serotonin reuptake inhibitors (SSRIs) and atypical antipsychotics that were introduced towards the end of the twentieth century.

The most obvious and prolific example of the psychiatrisation of everyday life has been through the proliferation of the drug fluoxetine hydrochloride (Prozac). Prozac, the first SSRI is prescribed for depression but has become, alongside the male-impotency drug Viagra, a principal 'lifestyle' remedy. That is, just as Viagra has been used to boost male sexual prowess (rather than merely to address sexual dysfunction), so Prozac has become a 'mind-altering' chemical used to combat the pressures and disappointments of ordinary human existence. Peter Kramer, an American professor of psychiatry, champions Prozac as a 'personality improver'. Just as Viagra is projected as providing men (and possibly women) with extravagant orgasms, Kramer argues that taking Prozac can make all of us feel 'better than well'. It is, for Kramer, part of 'cosmetic psycho-pharmacology'. However, unlike somatic cosmetic surgery, the SSRIs can be used not merely to restore, but to transform. Kramer highlights the transformative qualities of Prozac with anecdotal depositions from his own practice. The following extract refers to his patient 'Tess':

> Here was a patient whose usual method of functioning changed dramatically. She became socially capable, no longer a wallflower but a social butterfly. Where once she had focused on obligation to others, now she was vivacious and fun loving. Before she had pined after men, now she dated them, enjoyed them . . .
>
> (Kramer, 1994: 10–11)

Not only does scientific doctoring still prevail in the consciousness of the public as the dominant world-view with regard to health/disease, but the most irresolute area of medicine – psychiatry – is being seduced by the lush trappings of the scientific paradigm. The individuation of health/disease is increased through new technologies and drugs as the physician's gaze concentrates ever more intently on the internal organs of the patient. That is, the social and political environment is displaced as the search for disease converges on the infinitesimal within the human body.

Frank Furedi (2003) argues that an ever-widening definition of psychological distress and the manufacture of a plethora of mental disorders, along with the preparation of an army of psychological healers prepared to tackle any and all types of distress, has resulted in a 'therapy culture'. There is, therefore, an inflation of the importance of psychological distress and the need for therapeutic intervention – what I have described as 'therapyitis' (Morrall, 2008b). Moreover, no matter how loud and frequently the mantra of client-centredness and self-determination is asserted by therapists, for Furedi, clients are caught in an emotional Catch 22 situation by the very fact of receiving help for personal problems. Furthermore, as with Illich's point about medicalisation, therapyitis is not only disabling for the individual but leads to society becoming debilitated.

Alternatively, therapyitis can be functional for society, or at least for the powerful in society. Having therapy allows for 'emotional offsetting' (Tischner and Morrall, quoted in Morrall, 2008b). Emotional off-setting refers to the equivalent within therapy of 'carbon offsetting' within ecology. The practice of carbon off-setting absolves governments and corporations from guilt and the cost of damaging the environment. Industrial production, warfare, air and car travel can continue to proliferate and escape the moral and economic responsibility of significantly reversing climate warming, and clearing-up a highly polluted planet. George Monbiot (2007) argues that the planting of trees, erection of windmills, or attachment of methane-capturing equipment to the hindquarters of cows and pigs will not stop the catastrophic heating up of the earth. Similarly, therapy, whether indulged in through the use of self-help programmes and literature, or by acquiring a professionalised helper, does not stop the social causes of psychological distress. Neither carbon offsetting nor emotional offsetting can sort out the structural malfunctions of global society.

Structural sociologists, however, tend to view consumers as passive addicts, prey to the exploitative dealers in the production of medicalisation and healthism, dissemination into the public's consciousness and hegemonic indoctrination of medical ideas and technologies. But medicalisation is not all the fault of doctors or commercial purveyors of health/disease products and services. Although the medical profession and the merchants of healthism stimulate and feed the health/disease market with a never-ending supply of commodities, labels and promises, consumerist lust is also provoked by the public. People *want* pills, potions, incisions, and mind remedies, request to see their doctor for trivia, and propagate beliefs in medical infallibility.

Interactionist sociology judges consumers as not addicted but active in the construction of their own values about health/disease. They decide for themselves that it is meaningful for them to visit the herbalist or homeopath, or whether or not to buy an aromatic lotion to sniff, smear, or soak in.

The sociology of Anthony Giddens (1991) applied to medicalisation and healthism on the one hand and consumer demand on the other posits a reflexive relationship between the two. That is, the medical profession and corporations may set the agenda for what is considered normal and valuable concerning health/disease, but this is then distorted and reformulated by the reactions and demands of individuals. People do not follow blindly medical and commercial dictates, but have dictates of their own which may either produce accordance, concordance or discordance.

Giddens' reflexivity leads to the realist formulation about health/disease. Health and disease have a disguised reality and therefore conceptualisations about them will not be wholly consistent or fully predictable, but equally they are not wholly inconsistent or fully unpredictable.

Furthermore, of vital importance is health/disease in developing and underdeveloping countries. There is an argument for a realistic reappraisal of overindulgent medicalisation and healthism in the former parts of the world *and* a realistic reappraisal about under-indulgent medicalisation and healthism in the latter parts. Millions of people die from preventable and curable diseases because of the unavailability of (culturally sensitive) medical input. People in rich countries may suffer from iatrogenesis (along with diseases related to richness – especially coronaries and strokes). However, people in poor countries are dying from diseases that have already been eradicated or inhibited, or don't exist in rich countries (such as malaria, tuberculosis, HIV/AIDS, and Ebola).

There is, therefore, the need for a realistic approach to medical intervention. Side effects and errors are inevitable, as is some level of risk from new treatments. Doctors are expected to offer pills, potions, incisions, and mind remedies to alleviate conditions that distress their patients, and may have to make decisions on the basis of the better of two evils – either let the patient endure his or her torment, or satisfy a demand for succour by gambling that the cure will not be worse than the complaint.

Illich suggests that humans need to tolerate their afflictions, and that not to do so is reducing their appreciation of being at one with the natural world. Those who succumb to medical intervention are somehow ontologically substandard, implies Illich. However, the reality of pain and suffering from acne, cancer, childbirth, toothache, or depression mean that most people with these conditions would be quite willing to give up an element of their sovereignty to whoever wishes to administer relief and/or thwart an early death. That is, entering into the sick role is done by choice, and it is a judicious choice, given the circumstances.

SUMMARY

The issue of medical intervention in everyday life is one of paradoxical pressures and counter-pressures. On the one side are the related force of medicalisation and healthism. On the other, is first-world consumerism and third-world scarcity.

Whatever the pitfalls of medicalisation, the disciplines of disease by-and-large are attempting to help humanity. Doctors do contribute to reducing suffering and saving life. As Stephen Halliday (2007) writes in his book *The Great Filth: The War Against Disease in Victorian England*, medical practitioners along with midwives, scientists and engineers toiled as unsung heroes to prevent and cure such killer diseases as cholera and typhoid, as well as realistic social campaigners who attempted to alter the environmental and working conditions that led to early death. As far as is recorded, there were no postmodernist sociologists, unsung or sung, offering assistance in this battle.

Consultant cardiologist Keith Ball died aged 92 years in 2008. In his obituary there was a deserved respectful acknowledgement of his vigorous efforts to publicise the damaging effects of smoking cigarettes and persuading the Royal College of Physicians to do like-wise, and for co-founding ASH in 1971, the anti-smoking lobby group. He worked in the 1940s for the United Nations Relief and Rehabilitation repatriation of refugees from forced labour and concentration camps, and actively campaigned to have socio-environmental factors recognised as contributing to disease in many parts of the world (Kirby, 2008).

It is not so easy to defend the commercialisation of health/disease or to find such heroes as Ball within corporate capitalism or the consuming public. Bill Gates, founder of the ubiquitous and omnipotent Microsoft Corporation, may be an exception. Gates has given US$ billions to charitable causes (including large donations to the Global Fund, an agency set up to fight AIDS, tuberculosis and malaria (Global Fund, 2008)). However, money-making, not magnanimity, motivates Microsoft. Although the altruism of medicine can be questioned (as can that of the other discipliners of disease), there is no question that the motivation of the medical profession should be humanitarian.

FURTHER READING

Illich, I. (1975) *Medical Nemesis: The Expropriation of Health*. London: Marian Boyars.

134

MORAL ACTION

Be a hero: initiate or support a campaign against the spread of smoking in a developing or underdeveloped country (information about campaigns can be obtained from, e.g., Global Smoke-Free Partnership, www.globalsmokefree.com).

MADNESS

6

ROY PORTER, social historian extraordinaire (2003), suggests that there is a plague of 'mental hypochondria' in the world today. Certainly, madness seems to be proliferating, but are more people going mad, or is the prevalence of madness merely being recognised as hugely higher than the previously recorded incidence? If madness is at epidemic proportions, is it actually a bona fide medical condition or an interpretation of aspects of human performance that powerful groups in society deem deviant? If madness is a legitimate medical condition, does it stem from psychological and/or biological malfunction or from a mad society?

I am using the terms madness (and insanity) as a general term for the behaviours, emotions, and thoughts that humans have that become identified as medical diseases (or 'disorders'). Both the terms 'madness' and 'mental disorder' cover a wide and ever widening spectrum of human performance.

The World Health Organization (WHO) considers madness to be so endemic that if it is not already, it will soon be *the* most serious global health problem:

- Hundreds of millions of people worldwide are affected by mental, neurological or behavioural problems at any time.
- Approximately 877,000 people die by suicide every year.

- Mental illnesses are common to all countries and cause immense suffering.
- One in four patients visiting a health service has at least one mental, neurological or behavioural disorder, but most of these disorders are neither diagnosed nor treated.
- Mental illnesses affect and are affected by chronic conditions such as cancer, heart and cardiovascular diseases, diabetes and HIV/AIDS. Untreated, they bring about unhealthy behaviour, non-compliance with prescribed medical regimens, diminished immune functioning, and poor prognosis.

(WHO, 2008b)

Disease services for the mad are noticeably absent or embryonic in underdeveloped countries as well as in some developing countries. Many of these countries do not have policies, let alone services for the mad. In some developed countries where there are policies and services, these are chaotic. Across the world mad people have their human rights abused (WHO, 2008b; Morrall and Hazelton, 2004; Hazelton and Morrall, 2008).

Madness abounds in the overall disease-care systems of developed countries. Doctors and nurses deal with madness throughout their careers, meeting the mad in primary care, accident and emergency departments, and long-stay facilities. Branches of these disciplines, together with clinical psychology and psychotherapy, specialise in madness. Branches of physiotherapy, occupational therapy, and social work also concentrate their occupational efforts on madness. As with the rest of the population, one in four of disease practitioners will be diagnosed as mad.

It is unsurprising that because there are so many different occupations involved in madness, each with its own history, epistemological digressions, and internal conflicts, internecine strife within the mad industry (made up of consumers, workers, services, and systems), as well as profits to be made where the industry is privatised is rife. Notwithstanding this occupational tribalism, a de rigeur resistance to medical dominance by the non-medical disciplines, there is a general acceptance of the medicalised version of madness.

MAD PEOPLE

Defining what madness is, however, and what its boundaries are, and therefore who the mad are, is extremely problematic. To a large extent it depends on who is asking the questions. It also depends on what notions of normality are being adopted at the time, and whether or not there are identifiable behaviours and thoughts that are universally knowable and describable as to warrant the tag of madness.

Mad people everywhere are demarcated from the 'normals', as Erving Goffman (1963) describes those who have not been so categorised. This demarcation is either physical (that is, they are put in institutions that are either just for the mad or accommodate other demarcated groups such as criminals) or social (that is, they are excluded from living and working in the ways that the normals do). The basis for the demarcation is 'strangeness'. The mad are regarded as behaving and/or thinking and/or feeling differently from the rest of the population. This strangeness may be regarded as self-threatening or signalling danger to others. Individuals affected by strangeness might not be taking care of themselves (for example, neglecting personal hygiene and not eating), or could be suicidal or homicidal. An assessment of strangeness may be made by the sufferer (who asks for help from family, friends, or from 'professionals' such as the shaman, priest, or psychotherapist). Alternatively, assistance to become normal may be thrust upon those detected as abnormal by the agencies of social control such as the police, social services, psychiatry, and psychiatric nursing.

However, many normals hold beliefs, carry out actions, and have capricious emotions that are the same or similar to those of the mad. Suicide and violence are not confined to the mad. Non-mad people can decide to take their own lives, perhaps as a consequence of severe pain from a chronic illness, or a complete lack of hope in the future due to particular social circumstances. Football fans, binge drinkers, and young men, and more often than in the past young women are associated with a level of aggression that far outstrips that of most of the mad. Certain normals (for example, soldiers, police officers, and spies) are given licence by the state to kill in certain situations. Anyone (and there are lots of them) who considers astrology or tarot-reading to be truly predictive, arguably, is totally deranged. Richard Dawkins' (2006) and Christopher Hitchens' (2007) view of religion as nonsensical and dangerous implies that only the wildly insane could hold such beliefs.

Madness may therefore be just an arbitrary point on a scale of human performance that does not reflect a true partition between it and normality (Bentall, 2003). So why is there selectivity over who is condoned as mad when there is so much normal strangeness in society? There are essentially two interpretations that can be made about why certain behaviours and thoughts by particular people are deemed to be either so strange, or are of a particular type of strangeness that they merit an identity of madness. The first is that propounded by the mad medicine (and by association all the other mad disciplines). The second is in direct competition with the first, and offers social explanations of madness. While distinguishable from each other, neither the first nor the second interpretation is internally consistent. There are many disagreements between the mad doctors about what is and what causes madness, and what treatments can be effective. Likewise, there is a wide divergence of views from mad sociologists and other commentators on the social context of madness.

In general, however, mad doctors and their colleagues in the mad industry regard the mad individual as the locus for both aetiology and management, whereas sociologists argue that even if society isn't the origin of madness, then the way in which it is organised needs still to be taken into account in order to understand what might precipitate the condition and how it should be treated.

To add to the complexity of the subject of madness, however, some mad doctors deliver 'social' therapy through which there is an integration of personal issues with family and work-related factors. Psychiatric nursing, while remaining connected strongly to scientific medicine and empirical evidence, does have its gurus, some of whom are antagonistic to the medicalisation of madness. Moreover, a number of those who concentrate on the structure and culture of society in their search for the meaning of madness accept mental disorder as a fact (in the positivist sense). Others in the social madness camp deny that madness exists at all, but aim to supply remedies for the disabling effects of madness by exorcising stigmatising labels, and chastening those who do the labelling.

Perhaps the strangest observation to make on strangeness is that, despite the complicated and competitive definitional difficulties and terminology, both the public and the disciplines of disease would appear to 'sense' the difference that demarcates the mad from the normal. Such awareness transcends cultures and epochs. What is remarkable about the following abstract from the Reverand Francis Kilvert's diary, written from 1870 to 1879, is the ease of reference to madness:

Tuesday 4th July [1871]
Hannah Jones told me about the madwoman of Cwmgwanon. They keep her locked up in a bedroom alone, for she will come down amongst them stark naked. She has broken the window and all of the crockery in the room, amuses herself by dancing naked round the room and threatens to wring her daughter-in-law's neck. Then she will set to and roar till can hear her down the dingle at John William's house, nearly half a mile.

(Kilvert, 1978: 132)

Hannah Jones' actions are dramatic and therefore more noticeable and identifiable as strange. Much of what is sensed by the public about strangeness arises from more subtle expectations about what is normal. Schoolchildren and the media will use phrases such as 'nutter', 'bonkers', 'crazy', or their equivalents with equal ease as Kilvert did, but for much less flamboyant performances than rampaging around the house nude. However, culturally sensitised lay and medical diagnostic synergy should not be overlooked. That is, there is likely to be agreement more frequently than infrequently between relatives and psychiatrists about an individual needing 'help'. However, a nude rampage will probably result in 'help' being tendered far more quickly and assuredly than simply believing that the stars and playing-cards indicate the future, or that God exists.

Every society separates some of its 'deviants' from 'normals' on the basis of a perceived difference that does not seem to fit other categories of deviant human performance (such as criminality, drunkenness, impoverishment, religiosity, and 'new-age' lifestyles). Universally and historically, a discernible 'strangeness' in an individual's performance will attract a reaction. Whether it is called 'Amok' (Malaysia), 'Pibloktoq' (the Arctic), 'Bena Bena' (New

Guinea), 'Imu' (Japan), 'Koro' (China), 'Windigo' (native North America), or witchcraft (medieval Europe), the social deviance of 'strangeness' is being acknowledged and set apart from normality.

Demarcation will range from social segregation to physical segregation (although in some rural pre-industrial communities a demarcated individual may perform the role of highlighting and resolving *social* tensions: Helman: 2007). In the West, politically astute manoeuvring by the profession of medicine has resulted in the medicalisation of this strangeness. Psychiatrists, assisted by psychiatric nurses (and to a less direct extent clinical psychologists and psychotherapists) have been sanctioned as the arbiters of this form of deviance. They are the agents of the social control of madness.

MAD MEDICINE

The medical conceptualisation of strangeness as mental disease was already well under way in Europe by the time Kilvert came to write his diary, and eventually became the foremost explanation of madness in the West and is well on its way to prevail globally.

However, the medicalisation of madness had it origins thousands of years ago. Porter (2003) explains that the antecedents of medicalised madness in the West can be traced to the holistic explanatory schema for health and disease of ancient Greece and Rome. For Hippocrates and Galen, physical and mental health and disease were inter-linked. Humoral theory in particular (levels of black bile, yellow bile, phlegm, and blood needed to be in balance with each other to maintain good health) made both the body and the mind the province of medical practitioners.

Cultural beliefs, however, tend never to be wholly singular. The Greeks and Romans of the ancient world had their mythical and celestial beliefs coinciding with proto-scientific ones. In medieval Europe, mythical and celestial management of the mad, often mediated through such religious symbols as holy water, were customary and lasted well into the era of the asylum:

With those thought to be possessed, treatment was spiritual in intent even if it took a physical form. Belief in the power of holy water to cleanse the soul meant that lunatics were not infrequently bathed or suddenly ducked in a source thought to be holy. In the case of unexpected immersions in water, the procedure may well have been influenced by the observation that shock seemed to render some lunatics more sensible, at least temporarily. Other uses of holy water included the practice of blinding madmen and madwomen, sprinkling them with water from a holy source, and then leaving them to sleep.

(Andrews *et al.*, 1997: 102)

As Porter (2003) records, however, Christian, as well as Islamic, medicine in medieval times was interested in rationalistic ideas about both the body and the mind.

Segregation, although home-based, also came along early, as did the perception that seriously disturbed mad people could be dangerous. Plato advised that 'if a man is mad' (presumably this also applied to mad women), his family must not let him roam in the city to prevent injury to himself, to others, and to property (Porter, 2003). While those kept at home, if considered a nuisance or dangerous, might be tethered, kept in a pen or cellar, or, as with the mad-woman of Cwmgwanon, locked in their bedrooms, others roamed around the country during and after the ancient civilisations relying on begging and charitable and religious outfits for food and sometimes also lodging.

In the West, the profession of medicine wanted madness to be construed as disease akin to physical disease: in doing so, psychiatry was gestated. The version of the history of madness favoured by psychiatry is characterised by improved understanding of the causation, treatments that work, and humane care (Johnstone, 2000). Less attention is drawn towards the wacky management of the madness of King George III by the mad doctors, or the futility of spinning and dousing treatments so popular in the nineteenth-century madhouse.

By the late eighteenth and early nineteenth centuries, supernatural explanations of madness were being supplanted (but not removed altogether) by rudimentary scientific hypotheses about cause and treatment. Medicine, a rapidly professionalising occupation at that time, began to include psychiatry into its training courses, and to develop propaganda about its efficacy with regard to madness. Medicine portrays a world without psychiatry as one of mysticism, cruelty, and devoid of effective treatment and genuine compassion.

Medical historian Edward Shorter answers the question 'what was it like to live in a world without psychiatry?' thus:

> In Ireland it was like this: In 1817, a member of the House of Commons from an Irish district said: 'There is nothing so shocking as madness in the cabin of the Irish peasant . . . When a strong man or woman gets the complaint, the only way they have to manage is by making a hole in the floor of the cabin, not high enough for the person to stand up in, with a crib over it to prevent his getting up. The hole is about five feet deep, and they give this wretched being his food there, and there he generally dies'.
>
> (Shorter, 1997: 1–2)

According to Shorter's history of psychiatry, mad people received into the asylums were found regularly to be in a terrible state following years of ill-treatment at the hands of their relatives. One youth from Wurzurg had been kept in a pig pen by his father, and ate from a bowl by lapping up the food as would an animal. Many of those admitted into the asylums would have signs of having been beaten routinely:

> One [German] man had been chained by his wife to the wall of their house for five years, losing the use of his legs. . . . In England, such patients, if not chained at home, might be fastened to a stake in a workhouse or poorhouse.
>
> (Shorter, 1997: 3)

By the twentieth century, the medical profession had, once it had created it, taken over the mad industry so effectively that its under-standing of madness is accepted as the predominant operational basis for the policies of government and international agencies.

Psychiatry's understanding of madness is reflected in its classification systems. The mad doctors emulated their colleagues in physical medicine. Psychiatrist Jennifer Hughes extols the virtues of medical categories:

> A sound classification system is just as desirable in psychiatry as in other branches of medicine. Assigning each case to a recognisable

diagnostic category (while continuing to respect the importance of features unique to the patient concerned) has many advantages in clinical work.

(Hughes, 1991: 3)

There are two main classification systems. The first, the International Classification of Diseases, is compiled by the WHO. The second is the Diagnostic and Statistical Manual of Mental Disorders of the American Psychiatric Association. The fact that there *are* two systems of classification, and that both revise periodically their contents, implies that the psychiatric understanding of madness is not constant and universal. What is deemed indicative of madness may not have been so categorised yesterday and might not be tomorrow. Furthermore, the classification indexes have thousands of categories and subcategories of mind disease including: numerous types of schizophrenia, depression, mania, anxiety, compulsions and obsessions, personality disorder, delirium, psychosomatic syndromes, dementia, and difficulties with eating and body size. What is also included are: stuttering, stealing, frotteurism, voyeurism, fetishism, female orgasmic disorder, and male hypoactive-sexual-desire disorder. This comprehensive conceptualisation of madness indicates the degree to which psychiatry has colonised 'strangeness'. Potentially, any odd emotion, thought, or feeling will become the business of the mad industry.

Demarcation of normals from the mad through institutional segregation began in England in the thirteenth century when the St Mary of Bethlehem of London, a religious order providing care for the physically sick ('bedlam'), began to accept the mad. In continental Europe other institutions for the mad had been set aside for the mad by the beginning of the Renaissance in the fifteenth century. Around 6,000 mad people were incarcerated in the Hôpital Général de Paris in the seventeenth century, and subsequently incarceration of the mad spread throughout France (Porter, 2003). The 1845 Lunacy Act in England forced local authorities to provide institutions for the mad. A massive public building programme ensued and asylums housed more than 100,000 inmates by 1900.

The orthodox version of psychiatric history views asylums as necessary for the protection of the mad and to offer them a decent habitat and appropriate (for the time) medical treatment for the duration of their illness. Michel Foucault in his seminal work on madness *Histoire de la folie à l'âge classique* (1961) asserts that this is the age of the 'great confinement', and that the mad were henceforth debased to the degree of being rendered little more than wild beasts. There was, suggests Foucault, a 'great conspiracy' by governments and the propertied classes to separate reason from unreason. Industrialisation and capitalist economics required rationality together with order and diligence. Irrational undesirables (the mad) had to be removed from the gaze of the public. Segregated social control for madness began on a massive scale.

However, Porter challenges Foucault's proposition, arguing that apart from France, there was no 'great confinement' of the mad in Europe at this time. For example, it was not until the middle of the nineteenth century that the majority of asylums were built to confine the mad in England. Sociological structuralist Andrew Scull (2007) states bluntly that Foucault's ideas about the history of madness represents bad scholarship – Foucault got his facts wrong. Of course, Foucault's contribution to scholarship is to make the point that these are not facts, only ideas.

Although governments set the tone for physical segregation, the planning of and paying for confinement was not centralised, but organised locally. Moreover, although the Marxist notion that the mad were excluded from society because they were a patent reminder to the population of deviancy (their madness excluded them from adhering to a lifetime of being a cog in servicing the industrial machine and from servicing colonial expansionism by joining the military), it overlooks the fact that asylums were also built for philanthropic and humanitarian ideals (Miller and Rose, 1986).

Asylums in England had not been built either by or for the medical profession, but doctors were, as local notables, invited to oversee their administration. Institutional segregation of the mad provided a captive audience for psychiatry. Doctors could with impunity experiment with science and the inmates.

Asylums were forbidding and oppressive places in which mad people were committed perhaps for years, if not for life. Inmates were not just given invasive treatments but were habitually mistreated by their keepers, and sometimes by their doctors:

In 1812, scandal broke when Godfrey Higgins discovered in York Aylum (of which he was governor) thirteen women in a cell twelve feet by seven feet ten inches, and that the deaths of 144 patients had been concealed. The same spring, Edward Wakefield found a side-room in Bethlem hospital where ten female patients were chained by one arm or leg to the wall. In a lower gallery (traditionally the area of an asylum where the 'troublesome' and 'dirty' patients were kept), the pitiable figure of James Norris was found, confined to the trough where he lay. Norris died of consumption a few days after his release.

(Fennell, 1996: 14)

The New World was no better. In the USA the pattern was the same, with reports of mentally deranged people being kept by their families in cages, or in stables. Almshouses in Massachusetts contain locked rooms with inadequate ventilation where the mad would be put, sleeping on fouled straw. In Australia, the Freemantle 'round' prison housed the mad in tiny ill-lit stone cells.

However, this had not been the intention behind such massive financial investment in housing the mad, which could not be easily replicated today even in rich countries. Given the conditions the mad would otherwise have had to live under with their families or roaming the land, being inside an asylum with medical overseers may not have been such an appalling option. Having a roof over their heads with food supplied may have been some compensation for the physical restraint, cold baths, hot baths, rotating mechanisms, bloodletting, purges, and emetics, and eventually electro-convulsant therapy, psychotropic drugs, and psychosurgery they had to endure.

Some other types of institutions were built by contenders for control over the mad in industry in both France, the USA, Italy, and England. Lay benefactors and religious groups such as the Quakers wanted 'moral treatment' to replace the medically dominated asylums and physical methods of treatment (as well as cruelty). Moral management of the mad posited that an individual could be brought back to reason if he or she was handled more humanely:

This movement aimed in effect to revive the dormant humanity of the mad, by treating them as endowed with a residuum at least of normal emotions, still capable of excitation and training. . . .

They needed to be treated essentially like children, who required a stiff dose of rigorous discipline, rectification and retraining in thinking and training.

(Porter, 1987: 19)

However, employing a technique for occupational advancement which has served the profession of medicine extraordinarily well, moral treatment was introduced into the asylums alongside physical methods.

By the start of the end of the twentieth century, the profession of medicine monopolised the market in madness. Psychiatry was well established as a medical area of expertise, and madness had become as much a disease as lung cancer or liver failure. However, by the middle of the twentieth century a new threat was on the horizon – community care. The financial difficulties of continuing to operate huge institutions and a change in Western culture towards more tolerance by normals of non-normality meant widespread decarceration.

Community care might have meant the end of medical dominance because it opened up other approaches for caring for the mad and the input of other disciplines. Moreover, some psychiatrists turned traitors and, along with a few co-conspirators from psychology, psychotherapy, and sociology, rejected the orthodoxy of medical science and its physical methods. These anti-psychiatrists, a mixed bunch (if not mixed-up) of thinkers and practitioners, had their day in the 1960s and still hold a certain interest for some of those who are disaffected with medical dominance. Latterly, 'psychiatric survivor' movements have reignited the anti-psychiatry sentiment. From these sources, madness, rather than being a medical disease treatable with medical interventions, is considered a myth (Szasz, 1972), a label (Scheff, 1966), an understandable reaction to mad circumstances (Laing, 1960; Laing and Esterson, 1964), or a form of human performance that should be celebrated rather than obliterated (Dellar *et al.*, 2000).

The threat, however, was once again managed by medicine to its advantage. Psychiatry simply spread from the institutions into the community with its physical treatments. Community-based psychiatry (whether delivered by psychiatrists or general practitioners) was assisted enormously (as were the mad) by the discovery of drugs in

France and the USA that could dampen down psychotic symptoms. The power of psychiatry, and therefore the medicalisation of madness, has since been boosted considerably by the arrival of a new wave of psycho-pharmacological products at the end of the twentieth century, the development of sophisticated diagnostic technology, improvements in psychosurgery, and the accomplishment of the human genome map.

MAD SOCIETY

Sociological modification to or demolition of medical notions of madness stem from the realisation that it is either not a real entity or that is a real entity but is caused by society.

Structuralists in the main accept medical notions of disease, including madness. However, although disease exists, much of it is caused by or at the very least shaped by society. The maintenance of health and living a long healthy life (by not contracting disease in the first place) is also socially determined, as is longevity:

> [T]he social context can shape the risk of exposure, the susceptibility of the host, and the disease's course and outcome – regardless of whether the disease is infectious, genetic, metabolic, malignant, or degenerative. . . . This includes major afflictions like heart disease, Type 2 diabetes, stroke, cancers like lung and cervical neoplasms, HIV/AIDS and other sexually-transmitted infections, pulmonary diseases, kidney disease and many other ailments.
>
> (Cockerham, 2007: 1–2)

Of crucial importance, the stucturalist argues, are the effects of the social hierarchy on groups of individuals. The further down the hierarchy a person is positioned, the more debilitating disease he/she will suffer, and the earlier in life he/she will die.

People at the bottom of the social hierarchy suffer from madness far more than those at the top. This is so for madness overall, and specifically for alcohol and drug addiction, schizophrenia, depression, Alzheimer's disease, and personality disorder. There are a few types of madness, however, that do occur more frequently among those further up the hierarchy: eating disorders, manic-depression (bipolar disorder), and anxiety. Madness is also skewed by other structural factors such as gender, ethnicity, and geography (Cockerham, 2005; Rogers and Pilgrim, 2005; Coppock and Hopton, 2000).

The structuralist Andrew Scull (1979; 1984; 1992) refers to the role psychiatry plays as an agency of social control. Scull notes that generally it is the mad proletariat that psychiatry deals with, especially that large proportion of the mad industry that is state-sponsored. Scull posits that psychiatry serves the capitalist state by controlling the mad. The shift from incarceration to community care, Scull argues (wrongly in the case of England: Busfield, 1986), was purely an economic decision and had little to do with the discovery of new drugs or liberal ideas about human freedom. Drugs (and psychotherapy) are used to manage madness both in the community and within institutional facilities.

Social disorganisation theorists are also structuralists. This perspective considers the way in which urban areas are (dis)organised causes of not only criminality but also madness. Robert Faris and Warren Dunham's (1965) idea is that cities can be broken down into a number of 'concentric zones'. The specific characteristics of each zone either enhances, reduces, or increases deviancies such as crime and madness. At the centre of the city is the zone that contains the commercial sector, with shops, offices, small factories, and places of entertainment. The mentally disordered are represented disproportionately in this zone, which also serves as the sleeping and begging arena for the homeless, and supplies opportunities for a large amount of petty criminal activity. This today is also the area in many Western cities which is most heavily electronically surveyed, therefore increasing the likelihood of deviancy being observed and controlled.

Surrounding this innermost zone is the second zone, which is typified by slum housing, ghettos, and rented accommodation. Here reside new immigrants, the lower working class (semi-skilled and unskilled workers, many of whom are only partially employed), and the 'underclass' (the permanently unemployed, drug users and dealers, and prostitutes). If and when the members of these groups move up the social hierarchy, they have the opportunity to enter the third zone, which accommodates the 'stable working class' as well as former immigrants who are now more established within the social system. University students, attracted like other groups to the low cost of housing, reside in this zone in great numbers. When their studies are completed, most will move on.

Gentrification has taken place in segments of these three zones in Western cities with relatively young, either single or cohabiting, people who are without children improving poor housing stock or buying fashionably sited apartments (particularly near rivers, canals, or seas). Being close to a city centre offers the childless, young employed, and executives with a large amount of disposable income easy access for their work and entertainment.

Faris and Dunham's outer zone contains the residential suburbs. Traditionally, these have been inhabited by the middle class, but there is a growing trend for some of this group to reside outside the urban sprawl and travel into the city for work and entertainment, thereby creating 'dormitory' villages and new towns.

Faris and Dunham make the point that it is the physical environment that dictates how people perform (either as normals or deviants), not the other way around. Moreover, each area of the city keeps its identity despite the movement of groups through its parameters. Where there is significant population movement, there will be more crime and madness. The anonymity and social isolation that such population movements furnish will also flourish deviancy.

Added to the insights provided by Faris and Dunham is the observation by structural functionalist Robert Merton (1938) that communities and societies were 'strained' because of factors such as a rapid population turnover, warfare, or economic and political failure. Merton's concept of 'anomie' is used to summarise how people experience aimlessness, insecurity, and a level of despair that can lead to suicide when they are living in such strained circumstances.

The social disorganisation thesis and theory of anomie remains pertinent to global society in which urban living is now the norm.

There are other theorists who are not necessarily identified as structural sociologists but who criticise the structure of society. For example, Joel Bakan takes the view that global society controlled by large corporations is wreaking terrible damage to the environment and people for profit. Corporations destabilise the personal lives of workers by paying low wages, shedding jobs, and moving their operations if they find it financially expedient so to do or health and safety requirements become too stringent. Furthermore, for Bakan the ethos of profit-making has caused a pandemic of materialism, commodification, and consumerism on terms dictated by big business:

> Over the last 150 years the corporation has risen from relative obscurity to become the world's dominant economic institution. Today, corporations govern our lives. They determine what we eat, what we watch, what we wear, where we work, and what we do. We are inescapably surrounded by their culture, iconography, and ideology.
>
> (Bakan, 2004: 5)

This theme is taken up by psychologist Oliver James (2007; 2008). For James, sanity must replace the insanity of materialism of today's 'selfish capitalism' based on materialism and what he terms 'affluenza'. Much earlier than James and prior to the globalisation of capitalism, Erich Fromm (1963) argued that capitalist society was insane. Capitalism, for Fromm, is a type of social pathology akin to human madness because it contains major contradictions and irrationalities. These symptoms of insanity, he claims, have immense social and economic consequences. Wars are fought in which millions die to defend trading markets. Economic trading cycles produce periods of high unemployment and worker shortage. Mass entertainment, promulgated purely for profit, 'dumbs down' human culture and human relations. Life becomes meaningless and devoid of interpersonal intimacy.

Fromm could not have predicted the scale of humiliation for humanity that has now been achieved. Much of what is broadcast on television, printed in the 'gutter' press and in popular magazines, released in films and DVDS, and counts for social discourse on the Internet and through text messaging, is puerile in the extreme.

Viviane Forrester has also pointed to the madness of today's economic system. The discrepancies in contemporary capitalism have, she argues, engendered what she describes as an 'economic horror'. She suggests that volatile employment conditions have become the norm, and that this has resulted in a type of 'social hell' for those who are marginalised: '. . . look for instance, at a luxurious, modern, sophisticated city, Paris, where so many people, the old or the new poor, sleep in the street, their bodies and minds wrecked by lack of nourishment, warmth, care, also togetherness and respect' (Forrester, 1999: 28).

Interactionist sociology has come up with a seductive but ultimately disappointing labelling theory to try to understand madness. Labelling theorists do not accept madness as real in the medical sense. For example, Thomas Scheff (1966) proposed that medical madness was nothing more than 'residual' rule-breaking, by which he meant that this tag is applied by psychiatry when all other categories of deviance have been exhausted by the agencies of social control (for example, the police and judiciary). The interactionist Erving Goffman (1963) pointed out that there are serious negative consequences for such a label. Individuals so labelled become stigmatised and socially discredited. They have, for Goffman, 'spoiled identities'.

Thomas Szasz argues that madness is mythical, and that the practice of psychiatry is illusory. Szasz claims that psychiatry disables rather than enables its patients. People do not deal with the everyday issues of their life because psychiatry labels 'problems with living' as mental disease:

> It is customary to define psychiatry as a medical speciality concerned with the study, diagnosis, and treatment of mental illnesses. This is a worthless and misleading definition. Mental illness is a myth. Psychiatrists are not concerned with mental illnesses and their treatments. In actual practice they deal with personal, social, and ethical problems in living.
>
> (Szasz, 1972: 269)

For Szasz, medicine should stay away from 'problems in living' and only deal with conditions that have an identifiable organic origin. Psychiatric diagnoses are fabricated appellations attributed to 'symptoms', which may or may not have linkage to actual disease. The origin of, for example, schizophrenia may be found to be genetic, and other mental diseases listed in the DSM and ICD do have known biological causation (for example, the toxic states). However, most madness is not and will not be linked to organic dysfunction. Mental diseases, states Szasz (1993), have only the status of metaphor and should not be taken literally.

Szasz illustrates the fallibility of psychiatric diagnostic systems by exposing how they are constructed. He observes that the formal classification systems come about through a consensus being reached by a panel of psychiatric experts who make or break particular human performances as a disease. That is, it is opinion rather than an empirical observation of pathology that counts in psychiatry.

Szasz, as with Scull, regards psychiatry as an agency of social control rather than a genuine medical speciality. The state and psychiatry should be stripped of their powers with respect to madness. Psychiatry should leave misery, agitation, and bad and excessive behaviours to other non-medical disciplines. That is, people who have problems in living (and that would be most of the world's population in one way or another) should hire lawyers or psychotherapists to deal with these problems if they cannot sort them out themselves.

SUMMARY

There is a lot of madness about, but an agreed denotation of madness remains illusive. It does not reflect credibly on medical science that there is so much confusion about what madness is, and that the history of medicine involves professional opportunism and barbaric procedures. However, the continued upsurge in developments in technological investigative and diagnostic techniques, and psychopharmacological and psychosurgical treatments means that the medical scientific understanding of madness is strengthening.

Sociologists (and renegade psychiatrists) who promote the notion that madness does not exist contribute much to the understanding of madness, but do little to help the mad. To deny that madness is, no matter in what cultural manifestation, an agonising and (usually) unwanted experience, is as strange as the strangeness that attracts the label of madness. Madness is 'real' in the sociological realist sense. No matter what the cultural connotations, real people suffer from mental 'dis-ease'.

Medical practitioner and medical anthropologist Cecil Helman (2007) has reflected on cross-cultural variations and inconsistencies about madness at length. However, he concludes with de facto realist advice to other doctors when they are trying to understand what might be madness in their patients. After a complex coverage of theories and research, and the presentation of numerous case studies, the key feature of Helman's advice is that the doctor should be aware of the patient's culture when making a diagnosis of madness or should resist making such a diagnosis. He does not dismiss at any point in this advicce madness as a social construction.

FURTHER READING

Porter, R. (2003) *Madness: A Brief History*. Oxford: Oxford University Press.

MORAL ACTION

Help reduce social madness by carrying out one sane deed. For example, don't watch television for a week; ride a bicycle rather than taking a car for one journey; buy your next cup of tea or coffee from a small trader rather than a global corporation.

MISERY

7

It is proposed that happiness be classified as a psychiatric disorder and be included in future editions of the major diagnostic manuals under the new name: major affective disorder, pleasant type. In a review of the relevant literature it is shown that happiness is statistically abnormal, consists of a discrete cluster of symptoms, is associated with a range of cognitive abnormalities, and probably reflects the abnormal functioning of the central nervous system.

(Bentall, 1992: 94)

RICHARD BENTALL SUGGESTS (with such blatant irony that ironically he was taken seriously by some when he published his article in a respected medical journal), that happiness is a mind disease and misery an indication of mental healthiness. After all, in a world full of mess how can or why should anyone be happy?

More and more the miserable are obligated to find happiness. The blues must be replaced by rhythms of joy; the 'Black Dog' stroked until its tail wags; sadness replaced by joyfulness; negativity by positivity.

Moreover, misery has become a social deviancy that must be socially controlled. The general escalation in the surveillance and regulation of human performance is broadening across, and penetrating deeper into, moods. Happy citizens are good citizens. Miserable citizens are bad citizens.

Misery is a diluted form of melancholia. That is, the melancholic is merely more miserable than the merely miserable. Melancholia, refashioned as depression, has already become socially controlled through medicalisation. Misery is following suit, although it is susceptible to both medical and psychotherapeutic management.

When Robert Burton (1577–1640), English vicar and academic, first published *The Anatomy of Melancholy*, it was a bestseller by seventeenth-century standards and remains in print. Burton discusses with a Shakespearian literary flair sated with ironical mischievousness a state of mind that has now become the mind disease of clinical depression. Burton, while accepting the sorrowfulness and fearfulness of melancholy, pointed to the contrariness of melancholic mind-set. For Burton, self-diagnosed melancholic, the experience of melancholy is bitter sweet:

> Fear and sorrow are the true characters and inseparable companions of most melancholy, not all . . . for some it is most pleasant, as to such as laugh most part; some are bold again, and free from all manner of fear and grief . . .
>
> (Burton; orig. 1621; 2004: 67)

More so, the implication from Burton's intriguing treatise on melancholia, records Kevin Jackson, the editor of the 2004 edition of Burton's original and further writings on the subject, is that far from being a debilitating mind disease, it may signify intellectual and artistic genius. For Burton, melancholy may be distressing or enjoyable for the individual, and by extension, the same can be said of misery. Not only may misery reflect an appreciation of reality, but it can also be a prerequisite emotion for realistic action. Miserable realism is far more likely to lead to social change than deranged happiness.

The World Health Organization declaration in 1946 that the ideal human state was one state of complete physical, mental, and social well-being appears magnificently optimistic, but realistically it is dreadfully deranged:

> The famous definition of health by the World Health Organization as a 'state of complete physical, mental, and social wellbeing' is

... attractive. On reflection, though, it bypasses the unalterable reality of most people's lives, so the quest for such a perfect ideal of health is an equivalent form of madness.

(Greaves, 2000: 1576)

David Greaves (2000) points out that the modern madness of pursuing happiness obsessively is an addictive disorder. Psychologist John Schumaker (2006) comments that people in Western society are being conned into becoming 'happichondriacs'. General practitioners, psychiatrists, psychiatric nurses, psychologists, and psychotherapists are infecting the rest of the population with insanity by propagating the delusion, through the administration of chemical and talking remedies, that miserable humans can and should become happy humans. Moreover, there is a profitable and expanding self-help happiness industry selling happiness-creating products. Books, CDs, DVDs, Internet advice and programmes, specialist courses, and holidays on methods to perk up our mood abound. Such professionalised and commercialised attempts at mood manipulation are not only crazily unrealistic but grossly immoral.

However, the notion that humans should attain happiness stretches way back to the ancient Graeco-Roman civilisation (particularly Aristotle and Epicurus), and it was an important consideration for the Enlightenment theorists. Being happy is also an ideal for some religions (although most major Western religions prefer their followers to concentrate on suffering when they are alive and possibly for eternity). Happiness has also been not just a philosophical mantra but a political one. For example, the achievement of happiness is an absolute right enshrined in the USA Declaration of Independence (Bond, 2003).

However, psychological or physical homeostasis is not a fixed, permanent or desirable constituent of the human condition. Humans strive to improve their physical and mental performance, stretching and altering their prowess and acumen, attaining 'altered' body-and-mind states. Through such testing to and beyond the limits of former acceptance levels of human endurance and attainment humanity has progressed. Happiness, therefore, is not necessarily if at all what humanity desires or is functional for humans.

The nineteenth-century British political economist, philosopher, Member of Parliament, and utilitarian John Stuart Mill (1806–1873) wrote a great deal on the subject of happiness. However, he did not subscribe to the then accepted utilitarian view that the goal of society should be the greatest happiness for the greatest number of people. What Mill gave licence to was an acceptance of misery as part of the human condition, and a rather good part at that. Humans for Mill have talents far more lofty than those of animals which focus virtually exclusively on the fulfilment of basic needs. Once humans are aware of these superior abilities, they cannot find and sustain happiness if their talents are not satisfied: 'Human beings have faculties more elevated than the animal appetites and, when once made conscious of them, do not regard anything as happiness which does not include their gratification' (Mill, 2001; orig. 1861: 8). Moreover, for Mill humans should endeavour to use their intellect and morality in the struggle to understand and change the world. Only when their superior consciousness and conscience is utilised effectively can humans achieve happiness.

Mill linked individual happiness to a happy society. That is, unhappy humans would use their intellect and morality to make decisions which would furnish a fair and just social system. For Mill, only animals or human idiots and ignoramuses are happy with the satisfaction of base pleasures:

> It is better to be a human being dissatisfied than a pig satisfied; better to be Socrates dissatisfied than a fool satisfied. And if the fool, or the pig, are of a different opinion, it is because they only know their own side of the question. The other party to the comparison knows both sides.
>
> (Mill, 2001; orig. 1861: 10)

Mill also proposed that humans with high intellect and morality suffered the most. Moreover, the more consciousness and conscience are raised, the more misery escalates. Those who perpetually think deeply and constantly behave ethically will never gain contentment from only relieving their primary needs (hunger, food, shelter, and sex), but may also struggle to find any pleasure from ordinary employment and certainly not from what Eric Fromm (1963) refers to as 'dumb' popular entertainment.

So, with global society in the mess it is today, those people deemed to be happy can be considered stupid, mad, or immoral, a combination of these performance deficits, or all three. There is, of course, a contrary proposition put forward by the purveyors of happiness. For them, those people who report being happy occupy the cultural high-ground towards which all citizens of global society should head. Happiness becomes a goal in itself rather than as Mill argues an emotion that has no intellectual or moral authenticity unless all human problems are resolved and human civilisation has progressed as far as it can.

NUNS, RECTUMS, AND SLUMS

However, one stream of the happiness movement explicitly and superciliously regards itself as already occupying the authentic cultural high-ground – positive (or hedonic) psychology. Indeed, the stream of positive psychology, together with its bloated tributaries (the main ones being cognitive-behavioural therapy and 'happiness economics') has become a torrent.

Positive psychology originated in the USA, and its foremost authority is Martin Seligman, Professor of Psychology, at the University of Pennsylvania. Seligman, having invented positive psychology, has developed inventories and programmes from empirical (scientific) research to assess and improve an individual's happiness quotient in order to achieve what he describes as 'authentic happiness'. Authentic happiness the Seligman way means that an individual will be able to 'feel more satisfied, to be more engaged with life, find more meaning, have higher hopes, and probably even laugh and smile more, *regardless of one's circumstances*' (Seligman, 2008; emphasis added).

Seligman indicates that it is possible for most if not all people to obtain his version of authentic happiness. He's certainly made a good start. His website refers to the 700,000 users from around the world of his Internet authentic happiness course. Moreover, for Seligman where people live and how they live should be no impediment to such an achievement.

However, Seligman's notion of authentic happiness is not only far from Mill's belief that bona fide happiness is only possible once the circumstances of humanity have reached their progressive potential, but does not register as a feasible prediction with most sociologists because the point of sociology is that social conditions do affect if not determine human performance.

Nick Baylis is also a positive psychologist (or 'well-being scientist' as he describes himself). Baylis, like Seligman, accentuates the individual's ability to overcome his/her circumstances in the search for a wonderful life. Key to having a wonderful life is to learn from others who have had wonderful lives. Needless to say, he has published a book to this effect: *Learning from Wonderful Lives: Lessons from the study of well-being brought to life by the personal stories of some much admired individuals* (Baylis, 2005).

On Baylis' website, which advertises the lectures and workshops he can offer 'anywhere in the UK or Overseas' (there is also mention of his charitable and voluntary work), he defines what he means by 'wonderful lives' thus:

> By wonderful lives, I mean lives that are happy and healthy, helpful and good-hearted. A wonderful life doesn't mean a life that's trouble-free or without fault or flaw. It means it's wonderful that the person is still smiling and going strong after all they've been through. . . . Each idea is simply a tool that we can adjust *to fit our own circumstances.*
>
> (Baylis, 2008; emphasis added)

For Baylis happy individuals can affect positively their communities and societies no matter how negatively those communities and societies are affecting those individuals.

Such effusiveness about the individual being able to alter his/her circumstances is replicated by another positive psychologist, Tal Ben-Shahar.

> The goal of positive psychology is not only to overcome depression and negativity, but to ensure that every person has the tools to continue strengthening themselves in positive ways throughout their lives and be able to *access happiness from within.*
>
> (Ben-Shahar, 2008; emphasis added)

Ben-Shahar in his self-help book *Happier: Finding Pleasure, Meaning and Life's Ultimate Currency* (2007a) utilises the 'science' of positive psychology to argue that anyone can learn to be happy, or at least be happier than they were before buying his book. On his website he modestly states:

Tal Ben-Shahar

Teaching the World to Focus on the Good
(Ben-Shahar, 2008)

Apart from the global pedagogical function he has formulated for himself, Ben-Shahar refers on his website to his consultative role advising executives of multinational corporations, the public, and what he describes as 'at risk groups'. His campaign to teach the world how to be happy begins with 'happiness tips' (six of them). These tips involve individuals accepting that they are (only) human, doing things that are meaningful and enjoyable, appreciating that happiness is to be found in the head not the wallet, leading a simple life, taking exercise regularly, sleeping a lot, and eating good food, and being grateful to others who have been nice to him/her (Ben-Shahar, 2007b).

Providing tips is a regular feature of the happiness purveyors' promotional aids. Bob Holmes *et al.* (2003) have ten: earn enough but not excessive amounts of money; desire less; don't worry if you aren't a genius; make the most of your genetic predisposition towards happiness; make friends; stop comparing your physical appearance with others; get married; find a belief system; be nice to others; realise that growing old may not be as bad as you think. Richard Templar (2005), however, has a hundred, the first of which is don't tell anyone else what the tips (or 'rules' as he calls them) are, and the last of which is find yourself a new tip every day.

The purveyance of happiness, however, whether by tips, therapy, courses, or lectures, is not only devoid of any authentic sociological consideration, but, despite assertions to the contrary, is also scientifically shaky. Specifically, theories and techniques aimed at making people happy have emanated from subjective and idio-syncratic sources. Some of the happiness research seems to give credence to the accusation that it's not just the attempt to obtain happiness that is madness, as Bentall states, but the purveyors of this madness are mad themselves.

First, the weakness of the happiness scientific base stems from happiness research being 'soft' rather than 'hard'. That is, there is little or no objectivity in gauging who is happy and who is unhappy. Mostly, what people say about their own emotional condition is what counts as the primary indicator of happiness. 'Hard' data, such as mortality and morbidity rates, living conditions, and material advantage/disadvantage, unemployment/unemployment, and sophisticated technology (such as placing electrodes into the cerebral cortex and then scanning the brain), are used occasionally. However, even this hard science has to be conjoined with personal accounts of emotions, and rarely is situated within systematised sociological reasoning. Where attempts are made to be sociological about happiness, these tend to be trite observations and implorations about how some people manage to be cheerful even if they live in appalling places and have awful ailments, and how being cheerful may lead to these appalling places and awful ailments changing for the better.

Second, lessons about being happy are gathered 'scientifically' from small, distinct, and unrepresentative social groups, small orifices, or small countries and then generalised to the global population.

Nuns have contributed significantly to the establishment of the happiness bandwagon. The results from studies into what nuns do and how this makes them feel underscores much of the happiness literature. Although nuns are (usually) Catholic Christians, and stereotypically should therefore be riddled with guilt and anguish, some seem to have achieved nirvana, which is a Buddhist not a Christian concept. Nirvana for the Buddhist is the ultimate psychological state of harmony, peace, stability, delight, and contentment. The lifestyles of nuns are based on strict and shared routines. Nuns (at least those from Milwaukee) eat the same food at regular times, have the same access to disease care, conduct the same activities week by week, and do not cause researchers major headaches by introducing extraneous variables into their studies such as taking holidays, having wild nights out on the town, smoking, being promiscuous, getting pregnant, and binge-drinking. However, and this is why they have become so interesting to study, patterns in health/disease and lifespan vary considerably within nunneries.

Milwaukee nuns in particular are celebrated by those who have made their careers if not fortunes from administering happiness to the miserable. The School Sisters of Notre Dame, Milwaukee,

Wisconsin, USA took part in a longitudinal study. The research involved 180 of the nuns writing diaries about their everyday lives. This they did from early in their twenties through into old age (Danner *et al.*, 2001). Most of the nuns (nearly 60 per cent) exceeded their expected lifespan. Some lived way beyond their expected lifespan. The crucial dynamic at play in fostering a long and healthy life appears to be a consistently positive outlook. Put simply (and teleologically), old nuns are happy nuns and happy nuns get old. The nun researchers suggest that there may be an association between viewing life positively and living a long time because positive people have a different way of dealing with stress than negative people. In particular, they conjecture that positive people do not excite the release of stress-related biochemicals such as cortisol. Cortisol (popularly referred to as the 'stress hormone') can cause serious damage to the immune and cardiovascular systems and impair cognitive functioning if released persistently for any and every type of stress.

Rectums also appear regularly in the happiness literature (*Economist* Editorial, 2006). Daniel Kahneman, a psychologist and Nobel Prize winner for economics, and his colleagues probed their research participants' rectums for periods lasting any time from a few minutes to an hour in a Toronto hospital (Redelmeier and Kahneman, 1996; Redelmeier, *et al.*, 2003). What these researchers were trying to gauge was the relationship between the amount of time they probed a rectum and levels of comfort or discomfort reported by the proprietor of the probed rectum. The researchers were surprised to find that when asked about their experiences, the participants who had been probed for the shorter times reported a higher degree of displeasure than those who had been probed for the longest periods. The most significant criteria for the participants in judging their lack of enjoyment during the procedure were the 'worst moments' and 'last moments' rather than duration. A less painful end made the participants happier even if an end to the probing of their rectums was a long time in coming.

These rectal experiments, argue Kahneman and his co-researchers, show how memory is important for how people view pleasure and displeasure. However, it is the fallibility of human memory that is revealed in these colonic trials, they suggest. They conclude that what actually happens is not the important issue in the generation of happiness, but memories of events that become construed as having been happy.

From the probing of rectums the researchers extrapolate that people construct narratives about their lives (for example, concerning their relationships or careers) on the basis of momentous but perhaps momentary happenings. The peaks and finales are remembered above and beyond the totality of the experience. A love affair may be recalled as tremendously successful or a horrendous failure because what is retained is the memory of the periods of intense passion or concentrated exasperation. A job may be reviewed as having been a worthwhile element of an individual's life depending on whether or not he/she got the sack or was given a standing ovation at the leaving party.

American nuns and Canadian rectums are joined by Indian slums to add weight to the propositions of the happiness proponents. Robert Diener (2001) interviewed people living a squalid and impoverished existence in Calcutta, and compared their level of happiness with middle-class students from the same city. Astonishingly, the two groups were nearly equally satisfied with their lives. From the results of his research, Diener suggests that the important element involved in the attainment of satisfaction is the ability to find and maintain social relationships, again no matter what the circumstances. If an individual's interpersonal contact and community commitment is high, this will lead to high satisfaction about his/her life.

Diener also observes that a low expectation of satisfaction initially is also a critical aspect to how happiness is experienced. This indeed is a vital observation by Diener. Mill's realisation that a lack of education about human potential, together with the sociological insight that poor social circumstances are associated with a fatalistic attitude towards life, leads to a not outlandish conjecture that the slum dwellers made the most of their family and friends because they had nothing else to value, and that students could do likewise and take it for granted that they were also going to improve their lives. Hence, what needs to be investigated is not just what people say about their happiness, but their underlying motivations and expectations. Such research would have to employ far more sophisticated techniques than the interview.

MONEY, MEDICATION, AND PSYCHOTHERAPY

Apart from the nun, rectum, and slum studies, there is a factor that finds common agreement among the happiness fraternity and a plethora of social commentators external to that fraternity: money does not buy happiness.

Karl Marx (1971; orig. 1867) referred to the innate character of capitalism which requires humans eventually to become 'commodity fetishists', which then fuels 'conspicuous consumption'. For Marx, capitalism could only survive by expanding into more and more markets and by making people buy more and more things. In this Marx was accurate, but (as yet) his forecast that capitalism cannot continue expanding indefinitely and will eventually collapse and be replaced by communism has not (as yet) materialised. Far from capitalism collapsing it is communism (or versions of it that Marx himself is unlikely to have advocated) that is disappearing, and commodity fetishism and conspicuous consumption are becoming globalised.

Robert Frank (2000), Professor of Management and Professor of Economics at Cornell University, USA, has identified a new social disease – 'luxury fever'. By luxury fever Frank means that humans are spending more and more money on products that aren't necessary and do not lead to happiness. The novelty of big cars, wider televisions, and designer clothes, soon wears off. Further luxuries then are bought. However, like the drug addict, the luxury addict can only get a high for a while and has to go shopping again and gain. What Frank rather suggests is that people should work fewer hours and enjoy more hobbies.

Oliver James (2007), clinical psychologist and media personality, uses the term 'affluenza' to describe much the same social phenomena as Frank's 'luxury fever'. 'Selfish capitalism', another of his terms (James, 2008), is damaging to human happiness because it encourages people to turn luxuries into necessities and thereby foment envy about the possessions of others. Affluenza and selfish capitalism, argues James, rather makes people unhappy and has increased the incidence of mental disease. What Oliver wants is for people to stop being so greedy and relax, and for politicians to implement unselfish capitalism.

Social epidemiologist Richard Wilkinson and his colleagues (Wilkinson, 2005; Wilkinson *et al.*, 2005) postulate that although inequality globally correlates with life expectancy, in some poor societies people are both healthier and happier than their material status seems to warrant. Conversely, people in many wealthy societies are more miserable than their wealth would imply they should be. For example, the British, despite decades of unprecedented economic growth (and better health of the population overall), are as miserable today as they were in 1973 (*Social Trends*, 2008). The important variable here is equality–inequality. In countries with grossly inequitable societies, those at the bottom of the social hierarchy know that others in their society are much richer, and feel socially disrespected and suffer low self-esteem. In countries where poverty is rife but inequality is not, self-esteem is not affected in this way. What Wilkinson recommends are policies to raise social respect for all groups in society.

This disconnection between wealth and happiness is for political writer Gregg Easterbrook (2004) the 'progress paradox'. Rather than enjoying and gaining confidence from improvements in employment, health, intelligence, and material ownership, people 'catastrophise' that an economic or environmental collapse disaster is just around the corner. For Easterbrook, however, there are many reasons to be cheerful. What Easterbrook wants is for those who are living in abundance wherever they are in the world to stop whingeing about their predicament and be happy.

Other researchers have suggested that the paradox of wealth can be taken further. If money doesn't buy happiness, then could giving it away make people happy? This is what Elizabeth Dunn *et al.* (2008) concluded for their multi-method research examining the emotional effects of people spending their incomes on themselves and on others, as well as the emotional effect of winning large amounts of money. Although making money does buy some happiness, people gain more happiness from spending on others than they do on themselves. Therefore, they suggest, people should make a habit of generosity, perhaps only if this means paying for a friend's cup of coffee (all the better, of course, if it's 'fair trade' coffee).

Lord Richard Layard (2006) is the leading exponent of 'happiness economics'. Layard's happiness economics stems from the proposition that affluent countries have not got much happier as they have grown richer and that mental disease is rising. What Layard proposes is a mass programme of cognitive-behavioural therapy.

Layard's goal of making everyone happy may be laudable, but the means to achieve this goal (through psychotherapy) individualises what is a social problem: the mess of global society. Employing psychotherapy, especially the cognitive-behavioural type, aims to adjust the individual not society. Moreover, as Darian Leader (2007) explains, a similar form of psychotherapy to that of cognitive-behavioural therapy was used on the masses during the 1960s–1970s Cultural Revolution in China. The intention of the Chinese cultural revolutionaries was to alter the views of those who were suspected of stalling the full development of a communist state. Many of the suspects were not just (re)indoctrinated but beaten, and some were killed. This is hardly a recommendation for another attempt at readjusting people's opinions using a comparable psychotherapy.

For Leader, however, worse than the mass use of cognitive-behavioural therapy (and by implication positive psychology) to make everyone cheerful is the mass use of medication. It has been argued by Gordon Parker (2007), Scientia Professor of Psychiatry at the University of New South Wales, Australia, that depression is being over-diagnosed because the tools for measuring it have not been developed properly. The present threshold is too low, and therefore not only depression but misery has become medicalised. This argument does not imply that depression is not a real disease, only that it is not as common as the high level of medical intervention would indicate.

Leader (2008) explains that since the launch of the anti-misery drug Prozac in the 1980s, it has been prescribed to 40 million people across the world (and millions of others are taking similar drugs), thereby creating a multi-billion US dollar industry. The benefits and deficits of taking Prozac have been discussed ever since it came onto the market (Kramer, 1993; Wurtzel, 1994). Prozac therefore is being prescribed for misery as well as depression. However, Leader asks whether or not the Prozac bubble has burst. A meta-analysis of data on the effectiveness of Prozac report in 2008 concludes that prescribing the drug does no more to relieve depression than prescribing a placebo – given that a placebo does have an effect, and that Prozac still works for severe depression (Kirsch *et al.*, 2008).

However, Leader worries that cognitive behavioural therapy is being presented as an alternative for medication and is just as superficial in dealing with misery. For Leader, neither offers proper insight into the real cause of human problems. He is not advocating sociologically informed alternatives. He wants to replace cognitive-behavioural therapy as the mechanism for changing people's minds with psychoanalysis which, rather than digging deeper into the recesses of the sick society, digs deeper into the recesses of the unconscious.

With the obvious exception of Marx, what none of these researchers and theorists offer is a realistic means to mop up the mess of global society. Some only wish for such social change, while others want individuals to change through, for example, psycho-therapy or drugs.

BHUTAN, ICELAND, AND CYBERSOCIETY

If a structural change to society is needed to solve human misery, what does a structurally happy society look like? Are there real Shangri-Las in the world that exemplify a happy society? Yes, apparently, and the two most recommended as happy places to live are, first an isolated land of ice and second a Himalayan enclave (Morrall, 2008b).

The first one consistently wins the place in the world with the highest quality of life – Iceland. This is an under-populated, infertile, glacial island in the North Atlantic replete with geysers, volcanoes, springs, and Europeans visiting for a weekend of partying in its capital's bars and nightclubs or for a tour of its hot and cold watery attractions.

Iceland has no armed forces, is nuclear-free, and only became independent from Denmark in 1944 (previous to Denmark, the Nor-wegians colonised the country). Iceland's climate is wet and windy but relatively mild considering its geographical position. It gets the warming benefit of the Gulf Stream for as long as the Gulf Stream continues to be warm given the dramatic melting of glacial fields in neighbouring Greenland and the de-icing of the Arctic.

Iceland, therefore, is not an obvious place to find the ultimate in happiness. However, it does have one of the best standards of living in the world and an unsurpassed quality of life. This is because

Iceland has a 99 per cent literacy rate, average lifespan of 80.5 years, unemployment at only 1 per cent, high average income and a balanced distribution of wealth, a comprehensive welfare system, and social cohesiveness (Central Intelligence Agency, 2008a). Iceland's vibrant economy, made up of fishing, aluminium production, tourism and especially international financing, has provided the means for a happy society. But in early 2008, the Icelanders were jolted in their paradise because the economy, always vulnerable to the vagaries of the financial markets, seemed to be heading for meltdown (Dey, 2008). By the end of 2008, Iceland's economy *was* in meltdown, with its currency plummeting, interest rates soaring, and the Icelandic government requesting financial aid from the International Monetary Fund, the European Central Bank, the US Federal Reserve, and neighbouring countries, including Russia (McVeigh, 2008; *Agence France-Presse*, 2008).

Iceland's legislative assembly was established in 930, thereby making it the oldest formal proto-democracy in the world. Bhutan, on the other hand, only became a democracy in 2008, although it remains a kingdom. Furthermore, unlike Iceland it is impoverished. However, it has had a flourishing culture of happiness for much longer than Iceland and is much more obviously a Shangri-La.

Bhutan has institutionalised happiness by measuring social success using the 'Gross National Happiness' index instead of the economically driven measurements of 'Gross National Product' and 'Gross Domestic Product' which most other countries in the world adhere to. The 'four pillars' of Bhutan's Gross National Happiness are: (1) the promotion of equitable and sustainable socio-economic development; (2) the preservation and promotion of cultural values; (3) conservation of the natural environment; (4) the establishment of good governance (Esty, 2004).

This small and beautiful Buddhist country is sandwiched between India and China, with a population of over twice that of Iceland. The seventeenth-century Bhutanese national dress (the 'gho' for men and 'kira' for women) is compulsory. Smoking is banned throughout the country. Foreigners were only allowed into the country from the 1970s, and television from the 1990s. Tourism is restricted and surcharged heavily. Agriculture and forestry are the mainstays of the country's economy. There is free universal education and disease care. However, life expectancy is far lower than that of Iceland at 63.5 years. Infant mortality is heading towards 20 times that of Iceland. Literacy is only 60 per cent for men and 47 per cent for women (Central Intelligence Agency, 2008b). However, just as the Icelanders didn't expect their flourishing economy to become labile, so the expected result of the first Bhutanese democratic election, a landslide victory for the loyalist and very conservative Bhutan Prosperity Party, was unexpected.

The former King of Bhutan, Jigme Singye Wangchuck, and his son, Jigme Khesar Namgyel Wangchuck, who was crowned king in 2008, have tried to move their country into the modern world (for example, through introducing democracy) while maintaining the spiritual core of Bhutanese society. Having a conservative political party in power, no matter how loyal, was not necessarily welcome. Furthermore, the Bhutan state and the Bhote-dominant ethnic group received international criticism for discriminating against its ethnic Nepalese who are now either living in camps within the country or who are in exile in neighbouring countries (Morris, 2008).

Neither Iceland nor Bhutan is a viable model for every other country to follow, nor is it is safe to assume that either of these countries would welcome mass immigration by a global population seeking happiness. Not only are they different from each other, but both are very different from the majority of the world's major nations. Moreover, globalisation encapsulates and promulgates far stronger economic and cultural forces than can be mustered by less than a million Icelanders and Bhutanese. Furthermore, as Michael Bond (2003) points out, there are differences between countries that are fixed firmly within the globalising world in defining happiness. For example, in the rampant individualism of some capitalist countries such as Britain and the USA, it is personal achievement that makes people happy, while in more collectivist but still capitalist countries such as Japan, China and South Korea, not being happy is seen as a failure of society, not the individual.

If Iceland and Bhutan aren't the Shangri-Las they once were, could cyberspace offer a happy space to occupy? After all, the Internet provides a fantastic array of pleasure. There is a never-ending supply of networks, education, entertainment, and dating opportunities to keep people happy, and these are far more accessible than travelling to Iceland or Bhutan (unless you are already living in those countries, of course). What the Internet provides is the opportunity to improve an individual's social capital.

For Bill Gates, founder of Microsoft, the invention of the Internet has the same potential for human civilisation as electricity, the telephone, the automobile, and the airplane all rolled together. With reference to human interaction, he is equally as zealous about the Internet's magnificence:

> The Internet brings people closer together . . . communicating with a friend in Japan is as easy and cheap as communicating with a friend across town, and families regularly use the Internet to keep in touch with far-flung relatives. Millions of people with shared interests – no matter how obscure – exchange information and build communities through Web sites, email and instant-messaging software. The Internet gives people the opportunity to put their knowledge to work and take advantage of greater opportunities to lead productive and fulfilling lives. It is the gateway to vast amounts of knowledge, art and culture. It provides equal access to information and communications, allowing the formation of rich communities and forging real connections between people . . . It breaks down barriers between (and within) nations, opening up economies and democratizing societies. And as cheap computing power becomes more pervasive, the Internet can bring all these benefits to more and more people around the world.
>
> (Gates, 2000)

Cyberspace has, according to Nigel Edwards (2008), Policy Director at the NHS Confederation (and independent body for the organisations that make up disease care by the British state), had a revolutionary impact on human interaction. Computers and the Internet have aided innovation in medical science and in the storage of patient records. Moreover, he argues that the Internet is changing how patients and disease practitioners relate to each other. Edwards refers to 'communities of interest' whereby patients and their families share information and advice as well as forming lobby groups to demand certain treatments and services.

For Robert Putnam (2006), Professor of Public Policy at Harvard University, USA, acquisition of social capital is the key to happiness, and an element of social capital is knowledge about health/disease. However, Putnam is sceptical about social capital being nurtured in cyberspace. Virtual communities, he argues, do not replace the quality of real human interaction whether this is for entertainment, education, or networking, unless the outcome is actual human contact. The Internet remains a secondary consideration in disease care. Most patients for most of the time continue to have face-to-face contact with, and receive their treatments directly from, live rather than virtual practitioners, even if some enter those encounters armed with bundles of articles about their disease downloaded from cyberspace.

The exception, however, is dating on the Internet, as the point of this particular form of electronic communication is to have human contact of the most intimate kind, and to improve on one core aspect of social capital, a happy relationship. These extracts are taken from feedback supplied by satisfied users of one Internet dating site:

> Thank you! Really did find my perfect man . . . My experience on this site was positive, fun, and I met interesting, intelligent men that I wouldn't normally get a chance to meet in my social or work life. So goodbye from this blissful state of coupledom.

> Just wanted to say a hearty, shouty, very much meant thank you . . . we now live together, and we're very happy.

> [M]et my wonderful boyfriend on this site 6 months ago and now we are blissfully happy . . .
>
> (*Guardian* Soulmates, 2008)

This one dating Internet site alone states that it has 85,000 members. Another declares that it has 20 million members (Match.Com, 2008). A Google search using the rubric 'dating sites' I carried out in 2008 listed nearly 11,000,000. There are not 11,000,000 dating organisations, but there are probably thousands throughout the world.

Although it is not possible to evaluate accurately how many from these dating hoards actually find happiness, Putnam's scepticism is perhaps unfounded and Gates' suggestion that humanity should embrace fully the Internet as a revolutionary force for the good is not as mad as it once might have sounded, if only to find a mate with whom to enjoy a moment of deceptive happiness. Moreover, it is possible, although improbable, that patients will be happy to find their 'medical mate' in cyberspace. Through telemedicine patient and practitioner could engage in the equivalent of cybersex, thereby not even needing to turn up for a real date.

SUMMARY

Happiness is a duplicitous delusion. Promoting happiness or even being happy while global society and the physical planet are in meltdown is madness. To seek happiness when the world is in such a mess is immoral. The presence of deprivation, disaster, danger, and disease for certainly millions and perhaps billions of people in the world, seeking happiness or being told happiness should be sought is far less of a priority than trying to survive.

In the month that I was completing this chapter, BBC correspondent Claudia Hammond broadcast a report on the growing problem of cancer in Africa. She describes how in Ghana's second biggest city, Kumasi, she had visited a cancer clinic. This is what she found:

> There was just one nurse sitting at a wooden desk. But she was watching a black-and-white monitor, and there on the screen was a woman lying very still on a bed in a cell-like room. Broad tubes emerged near her feet from under the crumpled sheets. For the safety of staff, she was separated from them by several heavy, lead doors while she had the radioactive treatment. Still a young woman, she has cervical cancer, the most common form of cancer in Ghana.
>
> (Hammond, 2008)

There are only two such clinics and five cancer medical specialists in the whole of the country, which has a population of 23 million. Most people outside the main cities do not seek out scientific medical help but turn to traditional healers who use herbs.

Hammond makes mention of a charitable organisation called AfrOx which was set up by David Kerr following a call to action directed at all organisations: governments, international agencies, research bodies, global funders, the pharmaceutical industry, individual benefactors and NGOs made during the 2007 African Cancer Reform Convention in London. Kerr is Professor of Clinical

Pharmacology and Cancer Therapeutics at the Department of Clinical Pharmacology, University of Oxford, UK, and his multi-disciplinary team have a mission to improve cancer prevention and control in Africa using scientific medicine. They have begun in Ghana.

The reality of cancer globally and Africa in particular is spelled out by AfrOx:

> Cancer already causes more deaths each year worldwide than HIV/AIDS, TB and malaria combined. By 2020 there are expected to be 16 million new cases of cancer every year, 70 per cent of which will be in developing countries, which are least prepared to address the growing cancer burden. . . . Lack of resources and basic infrastructure [in Africa] mean that millions of people have no access to cancer screening, early diagnosis, treatment or palliative care.
>
> (AfrOx, 2008)

The young woman in the Ghanaian cancer clinic is unlikely to have survived by the time this book is published. On the day I wrote about her, fifty-one people in Iraq had already not survived:

> A car bomb explosion at a busy bus stop in northern Baghdad has killed 51 people and left another 75 wounded, Iraqi police have said.
>
> (BBC News, 2008b)

Furthermore, the 'science' underpinning the purveyance of happiness is somewhat dubious. The study of happiness has been exceedingly selective. Nuns, rectums, slums, Iceland, and Bhutan have contributed extensively to the setting out of happiness plans and principles. However, most of us are not nuns, do not take much notice of our rectums, do not live in slums or, if we do, then probably don't want to, and are unlikely to spend much time in either Iceland or Bhutan, if we visit these places at all. Moreover, relying as the purveyors of happiness do on subjective descriptions about happiness only produces skewed notions of authentic happiness.

John Stuart Mill's point was that he would rather be a miserable thinker than a happy simpleton. Mill also points to the immorality of concentrating only on individualised happiness: '[T]hat [moral] standard is not the agent's own personal happiness, but the greatest amount of happiness altogether . . . ' (Mill, 2001; orig. 1861: 11)

The removal of misery through medication and psychotherapy from the range of human emotions may lead also to the removal of empathy. Not to have experienced psychological pain (or physical pain) undermines compassion. If we haven't been miserable ourselves, how can we appreciate and act on the pain of others? That said, it is still possible to have some relief from the misery. This story by the late political activist Paul Foot may supply at least a momentary digression from the miserable message of this chapter.

Foot (2000) refers to a joke told by Gore Vidal about the former British Prime Minister, Harold Macmillan. Macmillan was visiting the then French President, Charles de Gaulle, and, during a meal with the President and his wife, he asked Madame de Gaulle what she was looking forward to on her retirement. The elderly Madame de Gaulle replied, 'A penis'. Macmillan naturally was taken aback but tried not to react as though this was an unusual retirement package. He did, once he collected his wits, respond with, 'Well, I can see your point of view, I don't have much time for that sort of thing nowadays.' Eventually, Macmillan was to realise that what Madame de Gaulle had actually said was not 'penis' but 'happiness' (Foot, 2000: 1576).

FURTHER READING

Singer, P. (2006) 'What should a billionaire give – and what should you?' *The New York Times* magazine, 17 December. Online at www.utilitarian.net/singer/by/20061217.htm.

MORAL ACTION

Contact AfrOx and offer to help.

SEX

8

H UMAN SEXUALITY, the gratification of carnal desire and/or the process by which the species is reproduced, is dynamic, elaborate, mostly pleasurable, and potentially very dangerous. It is dynamic because it appears to drive a considerable amount of human performance, and operates on many levels (including death: Bataille, 1986). Sex for humans is not just about making babies. It can bring potent psychological satisfaction and pungent physical release – if indulged in willingly, without abuse, and with some degree of skill. Sex, however, is also risky.

Disciplines of disease and students of health/disease need to know about sex for three reasons that are paramount to their work: (1) Patients are humans and humans are sexual, and therefore any claim to provide 'holistic' care by doctors and in particular nurses must take into consideration sex alongside other needs (although disease services in reality deal only with certain needs while over-stimulating wants); (2) some practitioners specialise in sexual disease, and most of those operating in primary care will have contact with patients who have issues about sex, whether this is related to identity, disease, or prevention; (3) disease care practitioners are sexual beings, and an awareness of their own sexuality and how turbulent sexuality is in global society today can help in their dealings with patients, if only to confront prejudice.

Moreover, doctors and nurses are associated inescapably with sexual stereotypes. Female nurses are portrayed in the media, pornography, and by the teams of women marauding around British cities drunkenly celebrating a pre-marital last night out, if not as virgin angels, then sexual libertarians, libidinous, busty, and adorned with starched aprons, black stockings and suspenders. Contrary media images present them as middle-aged, overweight, domineering, busty, but prudish 'matron' figures. Male nurses are stereotyped as effeminate, homosexual, sexually incontinent, and inappropriately employed.

Male doctors may have their public image moulded by the licentious, inept, comedic-tragic medical characters of films and television programmes such as *Carry On Doctor*, *Doctor in the House*, and *Doctor at Large*, or the maverick and sexually infused doctors of *M*A*S*H*, *Green Wing*, *House MD*, and *Scrubs*. However, as with nurses, there is the contrary image of the competent and sexually alluring 'Dr Kildare' type. Inexplicably, female doctors do not appear to have a strong public stereotype. Possibly, this is because the stereotype of a doctor remains that of a man.

However, sexually stereotyped, doctors, nurses, and the other disciplines of disease have perennially avoided dealing with the sexuality of their patients. Disease disrupts sexuality, but disease-care professionals customarily evade the question of how to compensate for the fundamental need for sexual expression. At best, lip service has been paid to the sexual needs of those people who have been hospitalised for lengthy periods (and sexual expression may also be a short-term requirement, especially among adolescents), those who are in residential care because of a physical disability, psychological incapacity, learning difficulty, or are elderly and infirm. No matter that the academic research and literature into the sexuality of patients and those in care is growing (for example, Wilson and McAndrew, 2000; Bywater and Jones, 2007), sex is an aspect of the patient's biological, psychological, social, and spiritual needs spectrum that is neglected (along with the 'social' component).

Such a state of affairs is stupid, but stupidity is common where human sexuality is concerned. In this chapter what biologists and sociologists have theorised about sexuality is rehearsed, some of which is remarkably stupid. Lastly, the wiser words of those with a practical understanding of sex and its risks are considered – prostitutes.

BIOLOGICAL SEX

> Boys are made to squirt and girls are made to lay eggs. And if the
> truth be known, boys don't very much care what they squirt into.
> (Attributed to Gore Vidal: Malik, 1998)

At the biological level, sexual urges can be simply about the
attraction that exists between men and women which leads to the
'mechanical' fertilisation of the female ovum by the male sperm.
Heterosexual intercourse, the insertion of the man's erect penis into
the woman's vagina, and the reaching of orgasm by the man, is the
biological mechanism through which the woman can become
pregnant (female orgasm not being necessary for the purposes of
procreation). However, even this obvious biological operation is not
simple at all, but involves a complex interplay of many factors such
as evolutionary pressures and the generation of sexually related biochemicals.

The external genitals and internal organs of reproduction,
facial characteristics, and physique, are decreed by biology. The sex
chromosomes we inherit (XX for a woman and XY for a man) provide a foundation for sexual identity. Secretions from the pituitary
gland following puberty stimulate the release of greater quantities
of specific hormones (in men, testosterone, in women, oestrogen and
progesterone), and produce physiological changes. For men, there
is an increase in body hair, growth of muscle tissue (arms, legs,
chest), lowering of the voice, enlargement of the penis and scrotum.
For women, there is the enlargement of the breasts, the growth of
pubic and axillary hair, the reshaping of the contours of the body
(shoulders, hips, buttocks, thighs) through the deposition of fat, the
broadening of the pelvis, alterations to the linings of the uterus and
vagina, and the commencement of menstruation. While interest in
certain aspects of sexuality is conceivable throughout infancy and
childhood (for example, a small baby may gain sensual feelings from
caressing her or his own genitals), fascination with sex is generally
unabated among post-pubescent youth.

However, evolutionary theorists argue that human sexuality,
particularly the difference between male and female sexual performance, can be explained in terms of the species 'reproductive strategy'
that goes beyond the release of hormones at puberty. Humans have

177

evolved a way of ensuring that their offspring have the best chance of surviving. This involves men having sex with as many females as possible, whereas women have a tendency towards mating only with one male. Male promiscuity and female sexual conservatism is designed, argue the evolutionists, to allow the man to maximise his potential to reproduce his genes through disseminating liberally millions of spermatozoa, whereas the woman has to conserve her resources and protect her genetic investment, given that she can only reproduce once every nine months. Thus, male licentiousness and capacity to carry out rape, and female sexual inertia and emotionalism, are reckoned to be integral to the process of successful procreation and the perpetuation of their respective genes.

Charles Darwin (1859), along with Alfred Russell Wallace (and later Gregor Mendel), laid the foundations of modern biology and genetics through his premise of 'natural selection' and the proposition of 'sex selection'. Darwin presented the startling idea to Victorian society that humans are animal and that animals (and therefore humans) are interested, in an evolutionary sense, in sex for procreation *and* survival. That is, animals will put themselves at risk from predators in order to attract a mate with whom to procreate. The passing on of genes is more important than the continuation of the life of that animal.

For Richard Dawkins, culture may also be passed on by the gene. He coined the term 'meme' to describe a unit of culture that provides some evolutionary advantage. However, evolution is essentially about biological, not cultural, manifestation and endurance. Dawkins' concept of the 'selfish gene' underscores the gene's overriding station in the evolutionary process: '[T]here is no difficulty in explaining the Darwinian advantage of sexual behaviour. It is about making babies, even on those occasions where contraception or homosexuality seem to belie it' (Dawkins, 2006: 194).

For example, male frogs latch on to females for hours if not days during mating (thereby ensuring that no other male fertilises the female). This puts both in great danger from agile carnivores as the conjoint amphibians are restricted in their movements and thereby cannot escape as easily as when they are not engaged in copulation. Thus, the production of spawn becomes more pressing than being swallowed by a snake.

There are, for Darwin, a number of essential components to sexual selection in animals that have application to humans. Male animals compete with other males for sex. This competition is won as a result of the greater physical strength, weaponry, and attractiveness (additionally in the case of humans, intellectual power, social status, and available resources such as property and money) of the victor.

> [Sexual selection] depends, not on a struggle for existence, but on a struggle between the males for possession of the females; the result is not death to the unsuccessful competitor, but few or no offspring. Sexual selection is, therefore, less rigorous than natural selection. Generally, the most vigorous males, those that are best fitted for their places in nature, will leave most progeny. But in many cases, victory depends not on general vigour, but on having special weapons, confined to the male sex. A hornless stag or spurless cock would have a poor chance of leaving offspring.
>
> (Darwin, 1859: 73)

The female is proactive in the selection process by making preferences about a mate, and the male (to some extent) is responding to her demands. The qualities of the preferred mate re-emerge in subsequent generations of the species, whereas the attributes of the loser are destined to become extinct. It is she who is deciding about the best stag or cock.

Evolutionary psychologists such as David Buss (1994; 2003) have taken Darwin's elementary concept of sexual selection and attempted to refine and apply it to human mating performance. In a multi-staged study lasting five years and involving fifty collaborators, over ten thousand people from thirty-seven different cultures across the globe, aged between 14 and 70, Buss reports that much of what he found disturbed him. What his respondents registered was a 'ruthless pursuit of sexual goals'. Mates are not chosen at random. That is, from this research humans appear as strategists. They humiliate and denigrate rivals, deceive and manipulate possible mates, and subvert their actual mates, in order to achieve their sexual goals. For the evolutionist, such apparently genuine and virtuous elements of human psychology as romance, love, and caring, as well as nefarious dispositions such as jealousy, rage, and emotional blackmail, contribute to the furthering of sexual objectives.

Conscious and unconscious mechanisms, allowing humans to adapt to all aspects of the physical and social environment, have ripened over millions of years. According to Buss, today modern humans have inherited the aspirations of our ancestors. In the days of hunters and gatherers, what a female required was a mate who could protect her during the long and vulnerable period of pregnancy and child rearing. She needed a successful supplier of food and heat, and a fighter to defend her from other males and dangerous animals. Therefore, women then, as today, desired men who could provide a stable and secure 'nest', and who could be counted on to be committed to a relationship and the offspring of that relationship.

In Buss's study, women throughout the world and across ethnic and religious groups, and in all social classes expressed a wish for financial collateral in a marriageable man. The trend by women to seek financial security was approximately double that sought by men. A powerful indication of economic viability in what women view as 'eligible men' is their high social status, or the likelihood (because of insinuated intelligence and ambition) of reaching an elevated position in society. Women wish to marry 'up' the social ladder, whereas men are much less choosy. Good physique remains on the sexual wish list for women tens of thousands of years after a large and muscular gladiator was needed to defend her from roaming sabre-toothed tigers and from being molested by (undesirable) men.

For men, youth is attractive in prospective mates as this is a patent declaration of reproductive capacity. Women's healthiness, another fundamental reproductive requirement by men, is indicated by, for example, universally recognised notions of beauty. Although the significance of a woman's weight varies cross-culturally, a standard waist-to-hip ration of 0.7 or below gives the impression to the perusing male eye that the target of his sexual inspection is not pregnant.

However, asks Buss, why should men bother to get married or commit themselves to a long-term relationship at all? To begin with, men who do not meet the demands of women may not have sex and procreate with the most desirable of females. That is, to guarantee their genetic prosperity, men have to agree to the terms of sexual mating as laid down by women. Furthermore, there may be an evolutionary requirement for a man to stay with the woman who has borne his children to ensure that they survive both in the physical sense and to pass on skills and cultural knowledge.

Interestingly, men appear to have an inherent reproductive technique to guard against another man successfully fertilising their partners. Women may be much more indiscriminate about who they have sexual congress with, and how many times they indulge in intercourse in order to get pregnant than is suggested by Buss's account of evolutionary processes. Robin Baker (1996) has argued that some spermatozoa have the specific function of attacking the sperm of other men inside the woman's reproductive tract. The occurrence of what he describes as 'the sperm wars' suggests that the biology of men has developed in response to female infidelity.

Far from adapting a biological-deterministic stance, Buss as an evolutionist is unusual in that he argues for change in human sexual performance. He concludes:

> We are the first species in the known history of three and a half billion years of life on earth with the capacity to control our own destiny. The prospect of designing our destiny remains excellent to the degree that we comprehend our evolutionary past. Only by examining the complex repertoire of human sexual struggles can we know where we came from. Only by understanding why these human strategies have evolved can we control where we are going.
>
> (Buss, 1994: 222)

The anticipation by Buss that humans can change is recommended as a way of coping with contemporary cultural problems related to sex. For example, our evolutionary legacy should not leave us unable to tackle rape, sexism, divorce, the 'sex war' between men and women, sexual disease, and human unhappiness in general. Social scientists have, of course, pointed out that both human cognition and the social environment have already altered the effect of biological imperatives.

Superimposed onto these biological impulses is the personal and interpersonal realm that in most cases mediates raw sexuality. Personal choice over sexual partners and forms (if any) of sexual expression, issues of self-awareness and confidence, the availability of willing partners with whom to consort, and the comprehension of what to do when the opportunity to have sex arises, influence our biological urges. Moreover, the high divorce rate, increasing numbers of single-parent families, growing appreciation of emotional and physical abuse in families, occurrence of infidelity, and proactive development of a single way of life ('singledom'), especially among young women, indicates that human mating is not only convoluted, defective, and painful for many, but also evolutionarily maladaptive.

This leads to an overwhelming criticism of evolutionary theorising (particularly of evolutionary psychology). Attempting to link aspects of contemporary human performance to historical conditions without any 'hard' or 'soft' evidence is mental masturbation of the most ludicrous kind because it becomes nothing more than teleology. That is, circular propositions are expounded as though they had a cause-and-effect relationship when all they ever can be are propositions.

That evolution has played and is playing a dynamic role in human performance and human culture, and that there is a biological effect on human sexuality is not in dispute here, only the stupidity of evolutionary psychology. However, overlaying both the biological and personal–interpersonal realms is the social (or cultural) domain. The norms of a culture or global society, while reflexively affected by the sexual innovation of individuals, can and does fashion dramatically the biological predilections and connotations of human sexual performance.

SOCIAL SEX

Gail Hawkes, in the 1996 first edition of her acclaimed book *Sociology of Sex and Sexuality*, wrote about the sexualisation of society:

> An ever expanding range of commodities is sold by invoking sexual imagery, while sexual desirability is increasingly presented as a leisure commodity to be acquired and utilized, whether in relation to self or others. We live, in short, in a sexualised world.
>
> (Hawkes, 1996: 1)

While some cultures continue attempting to exclude sexual exuberance, global society overall has become drenched in sexuality since Hawkes prophesied the coming of a sexualised world.

However, the sexual soaking of society has been happening over centuries (Foucault, 1985). One of the many peaks along a prolonged rising tide of sexual enculturation occurred in the 1960s throughout the Western world. During this period there was a liberalisation of attitudes in many areas of social life (for example, the arts, the press, politics, and the management of the mad). The 1960s sexual revolution came about in part because humans were for the first time in their mating history given the opportunity to free themselves from the risk of pregnancy. The invention of chemical contraception ('the pill') was followed by other mechanical devices aimed at stopping the process of fertilisation. Moreover, condoms became more easily obtained, and abortion became more available in many European countries and Japan as an unofficial (in some countries illegal) means of dealing with unwanted pregnancies. Pregnancy thus thwarted allowed sex to grow into a leisure pursuit. Former sexual 'deviances' were indulged by the media and the public to a greater extent than they had been for thousands of years in Western society. Homosexuality, formerly considered a crime and/or a mental disease, would be decriminalised and de-medicalised in many countries.

By the end of the twentieth century new global communicative technologies (especially the Internet) globalised trade, and international tourism had spread sexual knowledge, contact, innovation, and variation, as well as disease. The sexualisation of global society has been assisted by the profession of medicine along with psychotherapy, thorough medicalisation and therapyitis. Medicine and psychotherapy have formulated discourses and remedies for dysfunction in sexual performance, and sexual phobias and obsessions (Hart and Wellings, 2002; Morrall, 2008b), thereby creating specialisms in sexuality.

At this point sexuality began its second revolution in modern times, a revolution that continues today without a clear indication as to when or how it will end. As sexual practices transform, sexuality has entered a vacuum concerning performance and in particular morality. That is, the boundary between what is acceptable and unacceptable, legal and illegal, desired and expected, and who are the predators and who the prey, is yet to be resolved. The exception is where fundamentalist ideologies impose performance and moral tyranny, with what can be argued are either reactionary and inhumane justifications for the strict control of sexual expression (especially for women) or forward-looking and humane protectiveness towards vulnerable sections of society (especially for children).

Extensive capitalist commodification and the concomitant proceeds have been achieved by combining the selling of actual sex in various ways and using sex to sell a conglomeration of disparate products way beyond what even Hawkes envisaged in 1996. The sexual body parts of woman and men (in particular breasts and buttocks) and the sexual accentuation of other body parts (for example, lips, hair, eyes, and thighs) are used to sell cars, tyres, boats, computers, clothes, toothpaste, alcohol, shampoo, holidays, cigarettes, and, of course, cosmetics. Sex itself is sold through the explicit imagery that pervades cyberspace, popular magazines, and the pay-per-view television channels of hotel chains. Unless very effective 'filters' are used, any user of the Internet is vulnerable to frank advertisements describing how one's penis or vagina can be made-to-fit or expand/contract on demand. An 'erotic' genre is offered by many sellers of books and DVDs. It is hard to find a book, film, or television programme without a 'sexual interest' storyline.

In some European, North American, and Australasian cities, prostitution has become legalised or tolerated, and both 'soft' and 'hard' sexual accoutrements are sold openly in pharmacies and supermarkets. Viagra and its competitors are widely available on prescription, 'under-the-counter' in nightclubs, and through licensed and unlicensed Internet sites. Adults of any age are expected to be sexual. Having a 'sex life' in middle age through to old age is not any more regarded as perhaps unnecessary and unwelcome, or unavailable if wanted, and abhorrent by younger people. The message that 'sex is for life' not just for one's youth is actively promoted by the health police, and there is an associated commercialisation of lifelong sexuality.

Sexual desire and desirability are no longer alluded to within the 'dance of love' but declaimed. For example, in the prolific Internet arena of 'cyber-dating' and 'cyber-mating', it is usual for those advertising for a mate to mention aspects of their sexual proclivity.

Owning erotic implements is no longer frowned upon or a no-go conversational topic. Tens of millions of vibrators and other sex toys are sold each year globally, and together with pornography generate an industry worth tens of billions of US dollars annually. Starring in pornographic films (using, for example, cheap and widely available 'webcam' video equipment) is becoming an amateur leisure pursuit, with tens of thousands of such recordings occupying cyberspace. Some of these amateurs, such as 59-year-old Francesca, decide that showing their sexuality is worthy of a career:

> Francesca, 59, lives in rural Oxfordshire and is one of the UK's most popular Internet porn stars. She has her own website and is known as a BBW – a big, beautiful woman. She charges £15 a month for access to erotic photos and film footage of herself having sex with subscribers. Married for 33 years, she got into the industry when her husband and son died in quick succession seven years ago. While it was a painful period for her, being a widow gave her a new-found freedom.
>
> (BBC News, 2005)

As porn-star Francesca indicates, women are gaining sexual confidence. Nancy Friday is an arch proponent for the need to acknowledge and understand women's sexual desires. Her commercially successful books about female fantasies as told to her by respondents who replied to a request for details about what women day-dream about caused much controversy when they were first published. However, Jill Tweedie, one of the foremost British feminists of the twentieth century, novelist, and journalist, has a foreword to Friday's (1976) sexually explicit book *My Secret Garden*. In this foreword, Tweedie remarks that Friday's book, apart from being very erotic, is both fascinating and energising. For Tweedie, women's sexual imagination had been, up until Friday's book was published, 'laid underground', and is a dramatic provocation to male assumptions that women (unless they are nymphomaniacs or prostitutes) 'lie back and think of England' (or whatever country their lying happens to be taking place) when engaged in sexual activity.

In a later book, *Women on Top*, Friday lays the blame squarely on male sexism and patriarchy for the historical stifling of women's sexuality:

It was a patriarchal society that needed, for its establishment and survival, to believe in male sexual supremacy, or more exactly, women's asexuality. How could man wage his wars, put his shoulder to the industrial wheel if half his brain feared that he was being cuckolded, that the little woman was at home – or worse, not at home – satisfying her insatiable lust?

(Friday, 1991: 9)

Sexual contentment for both men and women has become a goal similar to the attainment of love, good employment, and wealth. Sexual knowledge is no longer confined to a few pages in an anatomy and physiology textbook, or to the 'top shelf' pornographic magazines. Nor does it rely on the very unreliable method of 'word of mouth' initiated in the school playground. Thousands of sex manuals have been produced describing and illustrating the best techniques for gaining more from sex. Some of these manuals are comprehensive in their content with regard to sexuality, and go far beyond simply instructing the reader on how to achieve, or give, an orgasm. For example, in *The Guide To Getting It On*, written by Paul Joannides and illustrated by Daerick Gross (1999), the following subjects are covered: kissing; nakedness; massage; male and female genitals; self-eroticism and mutual masturbation; sexual intercourse; anal eroticism; vibrators and dildos; talking about sex to a partner; sexual fantasies and dreams; having sex if you are disabled; sex during and after pregnancy; birth control and sexual disease; circumcision; impotency; cross-cultural views on sex; sex on the side of the road.

The sex manual industry is no doubt part of the commodification of sexuality and a cultural edifice of the Western world. However, other cultures have produced explicit guides to sex (for example, the *Karma Sutra*) in the past. Moreover, the display of sexuality and intricate detailing of sexual practices is a sign of the tremendous movement in cultural norms since the Victorian period.

Sexuality in Western society has moved emphatically from procreation (having sex to have babies) to recreation (enjoying the pleasures of sex for their own sake), and global society is going the same way. Moreover, there are now a multitude of sexualities: heterosexuality; bisexuality; homosexuality/lesbianism; transsexuality and intersexuality; and metrosexuality. Furthermore, sexual abstinence and virginity are making a comeback, and gay and lesbian people are getting married.

Masturbation for men and women is now considered not only normal but healthy. Sexual practices such as cunnilingus, fellatio, 'swinging', anal sex (heterosexual and homosexual), and sado-masochism (bondage, whipping, and spanking) are no longer taboo. This is borne out by the proliferation of sex literature in bookshops, subjects discussed on prime-time television/radio programmes, and apparatus and lotions readily available in main-street sex shops and chemists/pharmacies to ease the passage of pleasure and pain from these practices.

The exposé of Max Mosely's sexual interests illustrates the shift in what is perceived as acceptable sexuality. Mosely, head of the *Fédération Internationale de l'Automobile* (FIA), who is also the son of the 1930s British fascist leader Sir Oswald Mosley, won his case for the invasion of his privacy by a newspaper. The newspaper, the *News of the World*, reported on and recorded a video showing him being pleasured from pain delivered by the five prostitutes he had hired. Awarding him record damages, the judge for such a case, the Honourable Mr Justice Eady commented, 'I decided that the claimant had a reasonable expectation of privacy in relation to sexual activities, albeit unconventional, carried on between consenting adults on private property' (Eady, 2008: 54).

Moreover, sex drugs such as Viagra are significant in the refashioning of human sexuality. That is, Viagra has a cultural connotation as well as a penile one. Taking a drug that allows immediate (that is, after about a wait of an hour) sexual engagement replaces the need for prolonged eroticised courtship, romantic dinners, and late-night coffee (all of which might take many hours if not months). Humans can be perpetually prepared for sex. Such preparedness moves mating further and further from procreation, and perhaps beyond recreation towards habituation. Humans no longer need to procreate or even have enjoyment during sex. Sex may become similar to the mind-numbing routines of other popular cultural activities in global society such as watching television and shopping.

However, Western society did not invent sexuality. What the Romans (and Greeks) did for us was to leave a whole host of sexual tracts and habits. Sex was also important for the ancient Peruvians, as can be seen by the large collection of explicitly erotic ceramics housed in the Museo Larco (2007) in Lima. These ceramics reveal sophisticated knowledge about sexual pleasure.

The clichéd notion that Victorian society was prudish and sexually repressed is contested by Liza Picard (2006) in her study of life in London during the years 1840–1870. She discovered a raw underbelly of salacious sexuality, at least in London. The city, with its much smaller geographical area and population than today, had 3,325 brothels and nearly 10,000 prostitutes according to police records for the year 1841. Pornographic literature was on sale everywhere except, for an unknown reason, on railway stations.

The Greeks and Romans discovered the clitoris and appreciated its purpose, but this knowledge was seemingly lost during the Middle Ages. However, it was rediscovered by renowned medical practitioner George Drysdale. In his book *The Elements of Social Science* (1861), Drysdale covers in great detail the anatomy, physiology, and pathology of male and female reproduction, venereal disease, and prostitution, along with discussions on poverty, Malthusian laws of population, and the political economy of the working class. On the clitoris Drysdale states:

> In the anterior part of the vulva is a small erectile organ, analogous in form and structure to a diminutive penis, differing however in not being perforated by a canal. It is called the *clitoris*, and is highly sensitive like the glans penis. It is probably the chief organ of sexual enjoyment [for women].
>
> (Drysdale, 1861: 64)

Drysdale is against sexual abstinence, arguing that it is natural and healthy to exercise every organ of the body. However, he does not approve of masturbation, referring to the 'baleful effects' of solitary indulgence. For Drysdale, masturbation wrecks health. He cites cases of adolescent boys spending much of their day 'exciting their seminal emissions' up to twenty times. Physical and mental exhaustion, emaciation, morbid shyness, and possibly idiocy and madness ('masturbatory insanity') may be the result of extravagant auto-pleasuring.

Whether through auto-pleasuring, mutual masturbation or (less likely) coitus, another locale of extreme sexual gratification has more recently been found and researched – the 'G-spot'.

Conjecture about if and where an area of the vagina apart from the clitoris can, when stimulated, produce an intense orgasm, has been brought to a climax. Gynaecological scanning has revealed that some if not all women have an area of tissue within their vaginas that is relatively thick, and this is probably the site of the G-spot. The researcher, Professor Emmanuele Jannini from the School of Sexology, Department of Experimental Medicine at the University of L'Aquila in Italy, suggests that women could request a vaginal scan to establish where precisely their G-spot is (Geddes, 2008). Scanning, therefore, could make the otherwise prolonged expeditions into the vagina superfluous.

Notwithstanding the sexual freedoms of the twenty-first century (and vaginal excavations), double standards about sexuality remain. Apart from the continuation of 'loony sex laws' (Green, 2004), which means that in some countries or some sections of a country nudity is banned even in a person's own home, and which make oral sex (either fellatio or cunnilingus) or anal sex illegal, and execute adulterers, social attitudes may be out of step with a country's legal framework. For example, Poland's Law and Justice Party Government before it was ousted in 2007 stated in its bulletin 'Right Turn!' that gay people were 'animals' and 'emissaries of Satan'. The Latvian Parliament around the same time refused to pass a law prohibiting employment discrimination against homosexuals. Discrimination is against European Union directives (*New Internationalist*, 2008). Homophobia is not only illiberal within the working environment, but if extreme can lead to beatings and murder:

Cabaret stars are planning to make a Band Aid style protest song against homophobia after another shocking gay murder – this time a pensioner on his way home from the pub. 67-year-old Malcolm Bryan, who worked in the entertainment industry booking cabaret artists, was found dead at the bottom of a stairwell in a block of flats in Portsmouth last week. His death is the third gay murder in less than a year.

(Shoffman, 2006)

There are also considerable differences between the major religions about sex. Judaeo-Christianity is conservative about sexuality, while most Christian leaders are not keen on the practice of sex outside marriage and the Christian right are apoplectic about it and abortion. The use of pregnancy prophylactics is condemned by the Catholic hierarchy and Islamic religious law can be excessively punitive on sexual transgressors. However, sex makes Buddhists happy:

> Buddhists . . . make sexuality a part of their religion. They view sex as an important blending of energies that helps with one's spiritual transformation. Many of their most sacred shrines and altars show pictures of people have sex, and they sometimes speak of finding god through getting it on. Here in the West, sex is also an important part of religion. Everything that's bad is at one time or another blamed on sex. You get the feeling that sex was invented by the devil himself.
>
> (Joannides and Gross, 1999: 386)

The consequences of freedoms, public displays of raw sexuality, may be to push further the boundaries of the second sexual revolution into a third revolutionary period whereby 'anything goes'. That is, all forms of sexuality may become normalised. How this will affect the 'self' in society or society itself is an open question. It may liberate further the self from the shackles of moral regulation or eventually lead to an era of sexual subjugation.

Foucault (1985) has argued that Western society is heavily committed to the surveillance and control of sexuality. For Foucault (1985), sexuality is yet another social construction. Western society's fixation with sexuality, argues Foucault, has been manufactured through the medical and the psychotherapeutic 'confession'. A confessional takes place whenever a patient/client 'confesses' his/her story during a medical encounter or a psychotherapy session. Sexual preference, performance, dysfunction, and deviances are revealed to the medical practitioner and psychotherapist. Sexual disclosure allows sexuality to be regulated.

The argument that sexuality is a social construction is an absurd belittling of the biological impulse behind mating. The physiological side of sex cannot be divorced from its cultural other side. They are intermingled and inseparable. Furthermore, Foucault's history of sexuality could not take into account the Internet, and his idea of the regulatory confessional looks absurdly misconceived today.

As Francesca the porn star demonstrates, the confession has moved way beyond the medical clinic or psychotherapy couch, and is no longer just verbal but visual. There would seem to be a rush to expose not only one's mind but one's body, and this exposure is not confined to a doctor or psychotherapist but audiences of billions, and is not time-limited but infinitely accessible. We have all become priests of the sexual confessional as well as having the opportunity to take the sexual confessional. Surveillance has been democratised and control dissolved.

There is no way of knowing how the sexual paradox taking place in *global* society between fundamentalist cultures and liberal cultures that results in a form of sexual apartheid with repression and oppression on one side and freedom and frankness on the other will be played out. Each side has its own social problems to which each is reacting. Alongside sexual freedoms and contradictions there is the exploitation of women and children who are enslaved and trafficked for prostitution, the sexualisation of childhood, underage/teenage pregnancy, paedophilia, and a huge rise in sexual diseases, both of old and new types. Alongside sexual repression and oppression is archaic paternalism, murderous retribution, and the misappropriation of a basic human need.

PROSTITUTES

Prostitutes know a lot about sex, much more than postmodern sociologists and evolutionary psychologists. Sex is their business. They are at the kernel of human sexuality, its pleasures, exploitations, and dangers.

Elizabeth Pisani (2008) in her book *The Wisdom of Whores* rails against much governmental and non-governmental input into the most perilous aspect of human sexuality, AIDS. The WHO (2008c) estimates the number of people infected with HIV or having reached the AIDS stage may be 50 million globally; 1.5 million are newly infected each year, and 4 million are dying annually from the disease. However, these figures are likely to be considerably higher because the systems of data collection are notoriously unreliable. Some governments, if they allow statistics to be collected and made available in the first place, may 'massage' the full extent of HIV/AIDS morbidity and mortality for political reasons.

Pisani, epidemiologist, journalist, and AIDS policy adviser and fieldworker, has a groundbreaking mandate for realistic action. She is a woman of deeds not words, but when she does use words her message is informed, graphic, clear, genuine, hands-on, and pertinent. Such an accolade could not be handed to evolutionary psychologists or postmodernists. Pisani agrees that social circumstances shape people's lives, including their sex lives. However, the sine qua non of decision making, argues Pisani, is not whether or not they are poor but whether individuals act sensibly or stupidly. In her work many stupid people seem to have come across her path. The stupid people (or, as Pisani more politely says, people are not necessarily stupid, they just do stupid things) include clients of prostitutes, NGO officials, and politicians. The stupidest things they do covers: not wearing a condom; not using lubricants for anal sex; using infected needles; and throwing billions of US dollars at the wrong people – schoolchildren, boy scouts, girl guides, and virgins, instead of the real at-risk groups such as gay men and those who sell and buy sex.

As Pisani observes, sex, like drugs, has the tendency to make even sensible people behave stupidly. Quoting a (female) friend, Pisani records the mind-muddling capacity of sex:

> [S]ex is about 'conquest, fantasy, projection, infatuation, mood, anger, vanity, love, pissing-off your parents, the risk of getting caught, the pleasure of cuddling afterwards, the thrill of having a secret, feeling desirable, feeling like a man, feeling like a woman, bragging to your mates, the next day, getting to see what someone looks like naked and a million-and-one-other things'.
>
> (Pisani, 2008: 127)

However, stupidity is not confined to the brothels of countries such as Indonesia, where Pisani carried out much of her fieldwork. Surveys of gay men (3,500) in Glasgow, Edinburgh, London, Brighton, and Manchester found that risky sexual conduct was more common among men who knew that they were HIV-positive status than among men who were undiagnosed or HIV negative (Williamson *et al.*, 2008). Astoundingly, those who had been diagnosed the longest were more likely to engage in risky behaviour than those who had become aware that they were HIV-positive recently.

In the Northern Territories of Australia, carers of people with
learning disabilities assist in the procurement of prostitutes.
However, as consultant psychiatrist James Barrett (2004) discovered
when he raised the ethical debate in Britain about patients using
prostitutes, the practice was very controversial. Barrett cites the case
of an elderly frail man living in a residential home who wanted to
hire a prostitute. His request caused a dispute between the staff of
the home, representatives from social services, the man's family, and
Barrett, which was unresolved before the man died.

The disputes about the ethics and practicalities of recruiting
prostitutes continued in the *British Medical Journal* after Barrett
published his account of this case. It remains an unresolved issue
within the medical profession, and in the meantime a basic human
need and human right is being ignored or mused over indefinitely.
How sensible is that?

There are other debates concerning sexuality that prostitutes
might be able to shed light on, and help in rectifying stupidity. One
of these relates to 'gender' (that is, the psychological and cultural
transitive constituent of sex identity). There is little more apparent
in society, as Helman comments, than the division between men
and women. In virtually every country in the world, and at virtually
every point in human existence, men and women perform differently. This is not to say that elements of human performance can't
be swapped, or that there isn't performance flexibility between men
and women.

This division extends to those who pay for sex – in the main, it
is men who pay for sex and women who offer sex for payment,
although, as Pisani recalls, male prostitutes (some of whom have
procured additional female facets) are common in Asia and South
America. It also extends to who is being exploited, female (and male
prostitutes) patently being used and abused physically by men.
However, male clients also are being used and abused, but financially
not physically. It is extremely rare for a female prostitute to injure
or kill her client, but prostitutes get murdered by their clients. In
2006, eleven prostitutes were known to have been murdered in the
UK alone by men (English Collective of Prostitutes, 2006).

The debate continues between sociologists and biologists about
how much gender is determined by 'nature' or 'nurture'. Helman
(2007) suggests that an individual's gender can be assessed on the

basis of four elements. First, there is the underlying 'genotypical' formation (the sex chromosomes). Second, there are the 'phenotypical' secondary-sex characteristics (physical appearance, and body shape). Third, there is the psychological aspect (an individual's self-perception and understanding of her or his sexual identity). Fourth, there are cultural perceptions (norms of society that place pressure on an individual to dress, talk, and think in ways that are regarded as appropriate to a sex role).

However, the content of and relationship between these three realms is not constant. Certain civilisations have tolerated or demonised male and female performances that in other epochs were viewed in other ways. In Elizabethan times, it was thought masculine for men to wear cod-pieces, thereby accentuating the size of their sexual organs. The performance of striptease has historically been considered a female craft for the delectation of men. Striptease by men in twenty-first century Western countries attracts huge female audiences.

In Graeco-Roman culture, heterosexuality was not given a higher status than homosexuality (Foucault, 1985). Men indulged in sexual acts with women, slaves, and boys. Pleasures of the flesh (eating, drinking, and fornicating) were thought to be vital human dispositions. Indulging in these hedonistic activities was believed necessary to appease the pagan gods. However, it was the loss of control during sexual encounters that men in classical antiquity feared, and hence they had to be seen to be dominant in their sexual relations. Activity was, for ancient Greek and Roman men, 'natural' and indicated virility (Hawkes, 1996). What they despised was such inert acts as performing fellatio and cunnilingus, and being penetrated rather than being the penetrator. It was not homosexuality that was decreed abnormal but being passive.

Until the 1990s in the Australian state of Tasmania homosexuality was a crime. 'Buggery' in England and Wales, whether it involved other men, women, or animals, carried the death penalty until 1861 (Hawkes, 1996). The willing participation by adults in certain sexual acts is no protection from the law. In 1992, a group of sado-masochistic homosexual men, who had in private whipped, cut, and branded each other over a ten-year period (none of whom suffered any permanent injury), were found guilty in an English court of 'Offences Against the Person'. They also lost an appeal to the House of Lords on the basis that it was not in the public interest for people to cause bodily harm to each other for no good reason (Geary, 1998).

Helman (2007) records how there are also discrepancies within the genotype realm. Sex chromosome abnormalities may result in hermaphroditism whereby both male and female constituents are present, Turner's syndrome in which there is only one X chromosome, or Klinefelter's syndrome whose sufferers have the combination of XXY. These conditions are very uncommon. Just as exceptional is a misalignment between an individual's genotypology and phenotypology, whereby that person's sex chromosomes do not correspond to his/her genitalia.

Radical feminist Kate Millett in her book *Sexual Politics* makes the following observation about the connection between culture and sexuality:

> Coitus can scarcely be said to take place in a sexual vacuum; although of itself it appears as a biological and physical activity, it is set so deeply within the larger context of human affairs that it serves as a charged microcosm of the variety of attitudes and values to which culture subscribes.
>
> (Millett, 1977: 23)

Millett argues that the unequal power relationships between men and women in society are reified in the sexual act. Men copulate with women with the domineering intention as they enact in other spheres of male–female contact. However, Robert Connell (1996) argues that there is not one male role that each man adopts, but many 'masculinities'. Hence, the feminist stereotyping of men as exploiters of women and contributors to a patriarchal social structure belies the divergent performance patterns that can be found among men. Some men subjugate women, but some women abuse men. Many men do not engage at all in this power struggle with women. Moreover, men from different social categories have very contrary role performances and may have more in common with the norms displayed by women in the same group than their gender counterparts from other sections of society. Moreover, Millett was writing before the ascendancy of the social phenomenon of the arrival of the female predatory sexual performance.

Alfred Kinsey's research into sexuality, which began in the 1930s and continued into the 1950s, was to produce a taxonomy of human sexual habits that demolished the Victorian and medical separation of sexual performance into 'normal' and 'abnormal'. He did not accept, for example, that people were either 'heterosexual' or 'homosexual' (Kinsey *et al.*, 1948; 1953). He argued that individuals may have heterosexual or homosexual experiences which are indicative of what they enjoyed, but these do not reflect a specific type of constitution. Consequently, Kinsey was in favour of viewing sexuality on a continuum, which may have heterosexuality at one end and homosexuality at the other. However, this continuum has branches that lead to forms of sexual expression that cannot be categorised as either heterosexual or homosexual.

His sampling of white American men and women was to cause outrage. What Kinsey discovered in his surveys was that not only were the unmarried people of white America pursuing diverse and regular methods of sexual release (from masturbation to bestiality), but well over a third of the male population at some time in their lives admitted to having had a significant homosexual experience. At least 17 per cent of women had also been brought to orgasm by other women. Nearly all men reported that they masturbated, as did a majority of women. Clearly, masturbation could no longer be construed as exceptional, unnatural, or unhealthy.

However, one inescapable biological fact that denotes specific gender/sex role performance is that women become pregnant, have babies, and in the main take on the greater share of caring for their offspring as well as the home. Although fertilised ovum can be placed in men's abdominal cavities so that an (artificial) male pregnancy can be created, and house husbandry has become a variation on traditional family life, these events are still novelties. Women are usually constrained in what they can achieve in the workplace and in their social lives because of their reproductive capacity. This doesn't make such biologically induced constraint any more socially tolerable, particularly within liberal-democratic societies, but it does explain why it happens consistently and is so problematic to change.

Another inescapable biological fact is that of Foucault's death. Foucault was fascinated by extreme sexual practices (such as severe homosexual sadomasochism) and their connection to death. For Foucault, such practices were liberating as they removed all of the social constraints that dictate human performance. Foucault's ultimate sexual pleasure and complete intellectual freedom came from dancing with death by engaging in what he described as 'suicidal orgies'. James Miller has recorded Foucault's response, while he (Foucault) was lecturing at the University of California in 1983, to an undergraduate student's question about the risks from pursuing freedom through sex:

> Who could be scared of AIDS? You could be hit by a car tomorrow. Even crossing the street was dangerous! If sex with a boy gives me pleasure – why renounce such pleasure? We have the power . . . we shouldn't give it up.
>
> (Foucault in Miller, 1993: 353)

Foucault died a year later from an AIDS-related disease. Stupidly, Foucault lost his life, and society a magnificent if masturbatory mind.

SUMMARY

Charles Darwin certainly had a brilliant mind, but he was ignorant about what would be the effect of efficient contraception on the yield of children by the physically and socially privileged. Those that are, in Darwin's words, 'best fitted for their places in nature' (the healthy middle classes) now have far fewer progeny than those he seemed to consider are less desirable in the evolutionary sense.

Moreover, Darwin was ignorant about 'designer sex' (and although a scientist of immense intellect, he may have been more surprised at the invention of 'designer genitalia' than he was about the geographical distribution and variety of wildlife when journeying for five years on the *Beagle*). New reproductive technologies and sexual performance-enhancing drugs, in-vitro fertilisation, surrogate motherhood (and possibly fatherhood), the cloning of human tissue, and Viagra, have changed the ways in which humans can procreate, and sex is becoming a habitual recreational pastime.

However, it is as stupid to suggest that sexuality is wholly a construction of society as it is to argue that sexuality is constructed only by biology. Human engagement with sexual pleasure is a cognitive and cultural imposition on biological predisposition, but does not replace that biological predisposition.

Furthermore, the inescapable reality is that men and women, no matter how they operate in a 'gender' role, are usually biologically distinguishable and usually this distinction is manifest. Moreover, although excursions into homosexuality happen, the vast majority of sexual encounters are heterosexual. Prostitutes, while providing all manner of sexual services to satisfy all manner of tastes, understand this.

FURTHER READING

Pisani, E. (2008) *The Wisdom of Whores: Bureaucrats, Brothels and the Business of AIDS*. London: Granta.

MORAL ACTION

Gain information about religious objections to the use of condoms, then contact an objecting religious authority and object to their objections on the basis that people are dying by the million from AIDS, and condom use can prevent some or many of these deaths.

DEATH

9

Oh death. Oh death. Won't you spare me over 'til another year?

(Traditional)

A NEIGHBOUR OF MINE DIED recently. She died from cancer. She had lived near me for 11 years, but I didn't know her name until she was dead. Another of my neighbours, a medical practitioner as it happens, explained that she died in hospital soon after it was discovered she had metastases throughout her body which had spread from a previously diagnosed and treated breast cancer.

Cancer kills nearly 8 million people globally every year, including over half a million from breast cancer. The WHO (2008d) projects a figure of 9 million people dying from cancer by 2015, rising to over 11 million by 2030.

However, deaths from cancer represent only 15 per cent of human deaths annually. Each year 60 million people die. You and I, all of our friends, family, and neighbours, every person we have ever met (and haven't met) who isn't already dead will die eventually from disease or just deterioration. There is nothing so factual than the inevitability of our demise. Moreover, the predetermination of our death means that we are all in the process of dying. That is, dying is not something that happens only to those who will do so within a particular period of time; we die continually, each minute heading nearer to our death.

Doctors and nurses wrestle with death throughout much of their working lives, and do so more than other disease-care practitioners such as healthcare chaplains (midwives wrestle mainly with life). The disciplines of disease care have as their collective mission the alleviation of human suffering. This is so in the Hippocratic oath, both the original and modern versions. Implicit in most ethical philosophies and guidelines compiled by the disciplines of disease is doctors' duty to preserve the sanctity of life. However, although within the original Hippocratic oath there is mention of doctors not carrying out abortions or giving anyone 'deadly medicine', preserving the sanctity of life poses an ethical dilemma. While doctors and nurses are directly involved in care of the dying, they aren't always actively preventing death, and at times hasten death. On occasions, the abatement of physical or emotional distress may actually lead nurses and doctors to actively or passively kill their patients, either as a consequence of iatrogenesis, neglect, or as a deliberate measure to end a patient's pain. The removal of treatment or food, or the administration of certain types and dosages of medication, may or will induce death. Such action or inaction, depending on the laws of the relevant country, may be legal or illegal.

However, death is not all it seems. To begin with, some scientists (i.e. those persuaded by the logical positivism of Karl Popper, 1959) may argue that not even death can be guaranteed. We may believe that people (as with all life forms) have always died, but, just as we cannot state categorically that the force of gravity, although it appears to have always worked in the past, will continue to make objects of any size drop to the ground at the same rate, death cannot be predicted (in the logical, positivist, scientific sense) for everyone who is living now or who may be born in the future.

Moreover, the notion that death is certain for all living creatures depends on how 'life' and 'death' are defined, and who is doing the defining. That is, there is at times great ambiguity, both in terms of how the biological state of an organism is interpreted, and what social meaning is attached to that organism's condition. For example, at what point in the growth of a foetus does it change from a bundle of molecules into a person? At what point in dying does a body change from being a person to a non-person? Should a woman who kills her baby either for economic reasons or because she is insane be judged in the same way as a politician who orders genocide? These are legal and moral questions.

For philosopher Peter Singer, moral issues concerning life and death need to be re-evaluated (1975; 1995). Humans, he argues, are (only) animals. Morally, all sentient animal entities (beast, birds, or humans) should be regarded similarly with respect to suffering. Humans with severe disabilities or diseases, and other somatic and psychological malfunctions that reduce their sentience, can be compared (morally) with animals having similar lower levels of sentient acumen. The decisions and reasons to keep such beings alive must be taken on that basis. For Singer, the killing of a non-diseased cow, pig, chicken, deer, or sheep for human food may well be more immoral than aborting foetuses with Down's syndrome, not resuscitating an infant who has complex heart disease, switching off the life-support machine of a young woman in a persistent vegetative state, or a doctor supplying a lethal injection to a man with terminal cancer, or allowing a demented elderly person to die 'naturally' rather than being force-fed food and given death-preventing medication.

Today's social norms, mores, and laws concerning death have been moulded for thousands of years, as have understandings of what causes death, how long humans should be expected to live, and when they should be allowed, if not encouraged, to die (Kellehear, 2007). As (global) society changes, so does death. However, a number of classic sociological-approach studies of death still have pertinence to death-related disease care and the development of global society. These, together with novel sociological insights, have been grouped in this chapter under the rubrics of virtual death and social death.

VIRTUAL DEATH

Adults and children are exposed constantly to death, but, unlike previous epochs in all parts of the world where most people died in their homes and therefore were quite literally on display to other members of their family, friends, and neighbours, the expiration of life in the twenty-first century is mostly, if not wholly, experienced 'virtually'. While death to some extent is a non-event in Western society today, barricaded as it is within the walls of hospitals, hospices, and residential homes, it is conversely also a perennial and ubiquitous occupant of public space.

Throughout history, death has submitted itself nakedly as an everyday occurrence globally. People died at home, on the streets, and while working. As Giddens (2006) notes, in pre-industrial society, many generations of a family lived in the same household. This is still the case (although it is becoming less common due to the effect of economic and cultural globalisation) for tribal communities in parts of Africa, Asia, South America, and a number of South Sea Islands. Death happens as part of normal family life, and is much more firmly linked with the regeneration of life than is the case in industrial societies. That is, in traditional cultures death is viewed as part of the life cycle. Moreover, death is not individualised to the same extent as in the West. The remains of the dead person are viewed as either materially or spiritually attached to those who are living. There is, therefore, an indefinite endurance of life.

In the agrarian and early industrial modes of production of the West, and in developing economic systems today, children have died young and in abundant numbers. Their 'over-production' is testimony to the grim reaper's fondness for youth:

> In most traditional societies the dead do not really die – at least, not in a social (or emotional) sense. In much of sub-Saharan Africa and Asia and in parts of Latin America, they remain as an omnipresent part of the lives of their relatives and an invisible member of the family. Their death as a member of society is followed by their birth into the community of ancestors. Here they remain forever, observing, protecting, sometimes punishing those who survive them.
>
> (Helman, 2007: 223)

However, the over-production of children in these societies has caused and still causes the death of a significant number of women. Giving birth was in the West, and remains within underdeveloped countries and some developing countries, a very dangerous life event:

> Every minute, at least one woman dies from complications related to pregnancy or childbirth – that means 529 000 women a year.

In addition, for every woman who dies in childbirth, around 20 more suffer injury, infection or disease – approximately 10 million women each year. Five direct complications account for more than 70% of maternal deaths: haemorrhage (25%), infection (15%), unsafe abortion (13%), eclampsia (very high blood pressure leading to seizures – 12%), and obstructed labour (8%). While these are the main causes of maternal death, unavailable, inaccessible, unaffordable, or poor quality care is fundamentally responsible. They are detrimental to social development and wellbeing, as some one million children are left motherless each year. These children are 10 times more likely to die within two years of their mothers' death.

(WHO, 2008e)

Adults in ancient and feudal societies succumbed to death at half the average lifespan of those now in the West. Moreover, most adults in the past did not die in old age (a category which in itself is unstable). Routine wars brought death to each village and town, but it was not until the First and Second World Wars, along with subsequent regional conflicts and civil strife, that such high percentages of the populace were annihilated. Since the twentieth century, it has been possible to bring about the death of whole stratums of society (for example, armies of young men; Jews; homosexuals; those Russians considered 'reactionary' by Joseph Stalin; the civilian populations of Hiroshima, Nagasaki, and Dresden; Ibo tribes-people of Nigeria; Cambodians during the reign of the Khmer Rouge). The machinery and technology of war can produce death on a mass scale over a relatively short period of time, or (with nuclear weapons) instantaneously.

The effect on those who have been caught up in death during warfare can be personally devastating and socially divisive (Morrall, 2006a). Soldiers, despite training in killing, can not only suffer psychological damage as a consequence of causing the death of other humans, but may also find that on return from their fighting they are rejected by society. A common theme of American soldiers who had fought against the Vietcong in the 1960s and 1970s was that they were marginalised by a society that wished to forget about such a military and political disaster. The fictional character of Agapeton Mandras in Louis de Bernières's novel *Captain Corelli's Mandolin*, an account of the defence of Greece from invasion by Italy and then Germany during the Second World War, expresses his realisation that seeing death in battle makes an individual feel different. Mandras has come back dishevelled and distressed to his island home from the front line. Aware of the impact of the many deaths he has seen during the campaign against the fascist forces entering Greece from Albania, he ruminates about how his relationship with his mother and girlfriend has changed: 'There is a veil between me and them. . . . I have been to war, and they have not; what do they know about anything?' (de Bernières, 1998: 140). The medical profession, as it does so successfully with so many other areas of life and death, overtook the care of soldiers suffering from 'battle-shock'. The medicalisation of soldiers' experience of killing was to fall into the category of 'post-traumatic stress disorder' (PTSD).

PTSD has also come to be applied to the secondary victims of murder. PTSD is defined in the American Psychiatric Association's (APA, 2000) Diagnostic and Statistical Manual of Mental Disorders (DSM-IV-TR) when a person has been exposed to an extreme stress (such has murder) in which both of the following were present:

(a) The person directly experienced an incident or incidents that involved actual or threatened death or serious injury to him/herself or to another person, or has been told about or witnessed such an incident(s).
(b) The person's response to the incident or incidents was one of intense fear, powerlessness, or horror.

For a diagnosis of PTSD, the traumatic event(s) has to be relived persistently through conscious thoughts, dreams, or 'flashbacks'. These can occur because of certain 'triggers' such as a woman passing the location where she was raped, or a man who has been beaten up coming across someone with a similar social identity to his assailant. On the other hand, a person with PTSD may 'dissociate' from the trauma consciously or unconsciously, not being willing or able to remember what had occurred. There is, in psychiatric jargon, 'psychic numbing'.

Secondary victims of murder, whether or not they are diagnosed with PTSD, frequently use the idiom 'devastation' when describing their lives after a murder. Their customary patterns of eating, sleeping, performance at school or work, interpersonal communication, and planning are disrupted, and may never return to what they once were. Given that the global murder rate per annum is heading towards one million (Morrall, 2006a), death by murder is not just personally disruptive, but is seriously disruptive to global society.

Most people in former times, however, died because of disease not warfare or murder (or old age). In the past, epidemics of particular diseases brought death, which, in relative terms, killed more of the population than any war to date. The Black Death in England, which had spread from the Far East to Europe by plague-carrying fleas housed in the fur of rodents, wiped out perhaps 50 per cent of the population in 1348. Overall in Europe over a third of the population (25 million) died. In the 1350s and 1370s plague struck again in Europe, devastating city-dwelling communities. Paris lost 50,000 of its citizens in 1437 to the *Yersinia pestis* infection, the bacteria responsible for the plague. London (1665–1666) and Vienna (1679) had further epidemics, which caused the death of up to 100,000 people in both cities. The plague continued to kill huge numbers in the eighteenth century (for example, in 1720 48,000 died in Marseille, and in 1709 300,000 died in Prussia).

While the plague killed hundreds of thousands of people in India during the 1900s, and still poses a health/disease risk in certain parts of Latin America and Africa, it has been controlled through the use of antibiotics. What the people of plague-infested cities had to suffer during the Middle Ages, however, was the brutish slaughter of loved ones, friends, and neighbours by a foe whose mode of conveying death was not recognised and/or managed effectively, thereby creating a further proliferation of deaths. Ironically, the killing of rats, rather than the offending fleas, resulted in more infection. A dead rat is of no use to a plague flea, so it will jump to the nearest and most numerous warm-blooded mammal – humans. The scenes of decay and pain as (in the bubonic form of plague) the headaches increased in severity and the lymph nodes of the groin swelled enormously, or (in pneumonic plague) the lungs filled with pus and the coughing became severe and unstoppable are hard to imagine. The bodies would then be transported through towns and villages by open cart to charnel houses for burning. Therefore, no one, no matter what age or social standing, would escape the spectacle of death in its rawest and most barbaric form. Unless on a battlefield, where the entrails and limbs of fellow humans are torn from their bodies and strewn all around in a bloody blend of flesh and bones, there is no similar parade of tangible death in modern times.

Paradoxically, however, death is today available readily for our perusal and entertainment as a consistent theme in the content of radio, television, and Internet news broadcasting. We may in the West, as Philippe Aries (1983) observed over a quarter of a century ago, be reticent to acknowledge death, talk about death, or admit to our own mortality. In his terms, it has become a 'shameful event', but death is no longer 'invisible'.

Since Aries' observation there remains a conversational taboo with regard to the dying and death of those with whom we have an intimate relationship, and concerning our own necrotic fate as biological entities. For example, the USA Oral Cancer Foundation (2008) refers to how talking about death and dying is 'the last taboo' in American culture. Talking about sex is no longer taboo. There is no other subject of conversation that causes more embarrassment than death and dying (sex having spectacularly lost its taboo status). However, there has been a major cultural shift in this 'shameful event'. The perishability of human corporeality is highly conspicuous in the age of global information.

Death is exhibited starkly in documentaries about murders, wars, famines, earthquakes, tsunamis, and car crashes. Newspapers and popular magazines fill their columns with categorical details of homicides, suicides, accidents, and obituaries. Visually and in narrative, the mass slaughter of men, women, and children is reported recurrently throughout the media. The butchering of political and religious adversaries in Northern Ireland and Algeria, and the genocide in Bosnia and Rwanda, were delivered to a mass audience of death consumers. We gaze at the dead bodies being brought out of buckled trains in Germany, shattered aeroplane fuselages over South American mountains, and motorway pile-ups in Britain. We observe impotently and passively as the victims of drought in Somalia, and floods in Mozambique, hurricanes in the USA, suicide bombs in Israel, aerial raids on the Palestinian territories, and roadside mines in Afghanistan succumb to death:

Woman soldier among Afghan dead: Four UK soldiers, one of them
a woman, have died in Afghanistan after their vehicle was caught
in an explosion. The woman, believed to be a member of the
Intelligence Corps, is the first female UK soldier to have died in
the country . . . The deaths take to nine the number of UK soldiers
killed in Afghanistan in the last 10 days. The Ministry of Defence
is not expected to name the soldiers until Thursday . . . Since 2001,
106 British soldiers have died during operations in Afghanistan.

(BBC News, 2008c)

We are treated to a steady diet of bloody mayhem not only in the
media, but also in historical exposés of 'great tyrants' and imperial
powers. In every high street bookstore we can read elaborate
accounts about, and view vivid photographs of, atrocities committed
by the Nazis in Europe, the Americans in Vietnam, the British in
India, the Japanese in China, Pol Pot in the Khmer republic, and
Saddam Hussein in Iraq.

The dissemination by the media of actual death, however, is
supplemented by the omnipresence of fictional death. No radio,
television, or theatre play (whether, drama, comedy, or opera), or
plot of a popular novel is complete without a death (and sex) scene.
Films and videos portray the gore of dying by gruesome means for
a death-thirsty public. Children assassinate thousands of video-
game and Internet-game combatants. Modern culture is saturated by
the commercial manufacture of simulated death. Death has become,
like sex, yet another commodity either in its own right or through
which to sell other goods.

These deaths are not experienced at first hand, however. The
presentation and consumption of death, either in its real or artificial
version, is mediated through the prism of electronic or documentary systems of communication. Death, therefore, has become
both sanitised and 'hyperreal' (Baudrillard, 1988). It belongs to a
contrived realm of motion pictures and literature. Although we may
see real death at some point in our lives, and will attend our own
death, the countless numbers of other deaths we witness are
experienced in a virtual world.

I attended my neighbour's real funeral in a real church and saw
her real coffin being brought in and taken away for cremation,
but I could, if her relatives had wanted to do so, have entered

hyperreality instead: 'Pay-per-view service at crematorium: A new 'pay-per-view funerals' service will enable bereaved friends and relatives to watch proceedings on their computer screens if they cannot pay their respects in person' (Morris, 2008). So far, to my knowledge, there is no equivalent hyperreal service available for the actual cremation or burial of the body. Real bodies still have to be really burned or buried.

SOCIAL DEATH

Death is a social occasion. By describing death in this way I do not simply mean that it is a time when people get together either to celebrate the life of the deceased or to mourn her or his death. What I am referring to is the manner in which society orchestrates death. For example, death is a social event in the sense that society produces the conditions under which people die, and loss of life is hastened. Each year there are millions of people who are killed on the roads, die from smoking and infectious diseases, are killed in armed conflicts, and are murdered. The totality of these can be affected dramatically either up or down depending on how a particular country or global society overall is organised. Moreover, death rates are structured by social structure. Higher rates of death occur in particular parts of the world and within particular sections of all countries. The orchestration of death by society is related to the issue of health/disease inequalities. That is, the well-established relationship between social structure and mortality rates demonstrates that being poor, living in bad housing, and being unemployed will increase considerably your chances of dying younger than if you were materially well off and employed in a job that is satisfying. Furthermore, global warming, caused by specifiable economic, agricultural, industrial, and population-growth social policies or lack of policy, also brings about the death of people who are exposed to its side effects, and may eventually result in the death of all sentient life.

Ivan Illich (1975) makes the point that the way death is conceptualised is related to the structures and beliefs of a society. Rituals, such as post-mortem examinations, coroners' reports, investigation by the police into 'suspicious deaths', mourning, wakes, cemetery dancing, the reading of a will, the making of a tombstone, burial in the ground, in a vesicle or on a pyre, and the satisfying of legal and financial obligations, are elements of the death event that are socially created. What rituals take place will differ from society to society.

Society's view on health/disease will also affect how death is conceptualised. For Illich, the profession of medicine has intervened in life (by medicalising such personal or social conditions as pregnancy, illiteracy, and madness), but is also responsible for refashioning death. Death has been expropriated by the medical profession in the West. Doctors have successfully replaced purely religious connotations of death, which in themselves had supplanted pagan beliefs. Illich claims that the notion of a 'natural death', at the end of a 'healthy life' which is supposed to occur in old age, is a medicalised ideal which has at its core the image of the doctor struggling valiantly with potentially fatal ailments. If death happens at an earlier age, then it is considered 'untimely'. Medicine is striving continually to readjust the conditions under which death occurs, and at what age life ends. In this sense, all deaths as medicalisation becomes globalised will be retrospectively reclassified as 'untimely'.

Moreover, Illich argued with great foresight in the 1970s that in Western society the notion of death as a single God-given or normal event that is the same affair for everybody was becoming reconfigured. Today, there are multiple types of death, and an individual must be seen to have died from a specific condition. That is, people can die from one of a variety of forms of death, depending upon which fatal disease is diagnosed, and in which medical situation the death takes place.

People now have to die of something – of one or more medical complaints. Moreover, they have to die somewhere – in a medical environment. This may be an intensive care unit, a medical or surgical ward, an accident and emergency room, operating theatre, a 'dying unit', or elderly care ward. If an individual dies in a hospice or residential home, or in their own home, he/she still attracts medical personnel and paraphernalia. The visiting general practitioner, community nurse or occupational therapist, along with the staff of the hospice or residential home, disgorges the medical discourse even into the private bedroom of the dead. Dying on the roadside does not mean escape from the tentacles of the medical profession. An ambulance crew or mobile paramedics will be hailed, thereby signifying a medicalised death.

A masterpiece study of the social organisation of dying and death within hospitals was conducted by Barney Glaser and Anselm Strauss in the 1960s. The conclusions from the interactionist approach taken by these researchers still have application in today's disease services. Glaser and Strauss (1965) produced a simple typology of communications that can be used to analyse more or less all disease-care situations. Whether in institutions or the community, communications are transpiring between the key players in the drama of death. Knowledge can enable patients and their significant others, and disease-care practitioners, to produce overall and individual policies on what should or should not be divulged about the disease status of the dying person.

The interactions between disease-care practitioners (principally doctors and nurses), relatives, and the person who is dying are seen to fit into one of four *Awareness Contexts* in Glaser and Strauss's research. The first of these categories is *Closed Awareness*. Here, the patient is not cognisant of her/his looming expiration. However, others (that is, the disease-care practitioners and the relatives) are. That is, the patient may understand that he/she is ill, and perhaps even realise that the illness is severe, but he/she does not comprehend fully that death rather than cure or living with a chronic condition is going to be the outcome.

The second context for Glaser and Strauss is that of *Suspected Awareness*. The patient guesses that others may know he/she is dying (and they do). Here both the patient and those around her/him are caught in a communicative quandary. For the patient, it may be better to have her/his suspicion confirmed or denied rather than being left in doubt. Hence, the patient may ask indirect questions to gain more clues, and these may be sought from people with whom he/she only has peripheral involvement, or who are junior members of staff. Alternatively, the patient may ask bluntly his/her doctor, nurse, or partner 'Am I going to die?'. For the staff caring for the dying patient and her/his relatives, the dilemma can be about whether or not to explain the reality of the situation if asked, or to give reassurance that this is not the case. Repudiating the patient's suspicions may be carried out in the belief that being aware of one's imminent death may increase psychological suffering or hasten death.

Such preclusion, however, may also be the result of diagnostic uncertainty. That is, medical opinion may be less than absolute about the patient's condition and the chances of survival. Consequently, the verification of a patient's prospects as hopeless, and then to find that he/she has not died, may cause both professional embarrassment and possibly a law suit filed against the physician and/or the hospital. Furthermore, for some medical conditions (for example, HIV/AIDS and particular cancers) new medical treatments are regularly discovered (although nowhere near as often as is reported by the media), and these may delay death beyond the expected point. A patient given a prognosis of only six months to live could find that a potent drug has been marketed during that period. The patient could then have the judgement of his/her life expectancy extended, and this may happen time and time again. In such circumstances, to tell a patient that death is assured might seem inappropriate ethically to the attending practitioners and callous to the relatives. Uncertainty here is not the result of medical-scientific fallibility, or communicative incompetence on behalf of disease-care practitioners, but due to the quirkiness of scientific inventiveness, and the bureaucratic complexities involved in gaining approval for novel medical treatments and procedures.

If the patient takes the course of not seeking confirmation of her or his suspicions, then according to Glaser and Strauss a third context may be entered, that of *Mutual Pretence Awareness*. There is, they suggested, a 'dying situation' in which everyone knows of the patient's condition, and the patient also understands that he/she has not long to live, but that all pretend that this is not the case. That is, there is an atmosphere of false hope generated from both the healthcare staff and relatives, and the patient. No one admits candidly what all know to be the outcome of contracting the disease in question – death.

At variance with the other three contexts, *Open Awareness* occurs when all the relevant players (including the patient) acknowledge that the patient is dying. The subject of death and the processes involved in dying are discussed freely. This may take the form of the patient asking for information from the disease-care practitioners about what pain he/she might endure, talking over personal issues with his/her loved ones, and/or making preparations for death (for example, settling financial matters). Of course, the patient may also become distraught, incapable of dealing with day-to-day activities such as eating and washing, let alone sorting out major issues such as their will and mortgage, and also obsessed with the ephemerality of life. That is, it should not be assumed automatically that *Open Awareness* is synonymous with patient contentment, nor that by taking this option all ethical predicaments in the care of the dying are therefore resolved.

In the situation of *Closed Awareness* there is not necessarily a deliberate attempt to protect the dying person from knowing his/her impending demise. Not telling the patient may be a way for the practitioners and relatives to avoid painful discussions on a subject that is not only distressing to them, but for which they feel inadequately prepared. That is, it may be that practitioners and the relatives are safeguarding themselves from psychological anxiety, as a consequence of the continued taboo status surrounding any talk about the real death of a loved one or our own death. A *Closed Awareness* context can therefore be considered as not discrepant with the conventional social norms in the Anglo-Celtic cultures of the British Isles, Australasia, and much of North America. Indeed, David Field (1989), who is in favour of more openness, nevertheless connects Western medical treatments and medical procedures to the practice of not telling patients about their ailments. That is, there is epistemological and practice consistency in the care of the dying because not being too open about anything concerning disease care is the normal communicative pattern.

Moreover, the structural and cultural complexities of society may mean that to operate outside of this context can contravene accepted patterns of behaviour for certain ethnic minorities, age groups, and social classes. It is also more likely to be the standard interactive pattern for men rather than women. Deborah Tannen's (1992) description of stoicism, independence, and achievement being male characteristics, and intimacy and sharing being female characteristics, suggests that the subject of dying may be more shut off from the former than the latter.

Furthermore, there is a tension between the social norms of either the dominant ideology of a society, or those adhered to by a particular subdivision of that society, and the practice of 'openness' increasingly advocated as ethical by many of those practitioners caring for people who are dying. This tension may be in part responsible for some of the ambiguity and apparent dishonesty that surround the contexts of *Suspected Awareness* and *Mutual Pretence Awareness*.

For example, Swiss-born psychiatrist and inventive writer in the field of death and dying, Elizabeth Kubler-Ross (1969), has had a huge influence on how dying and death are dealt with by disease-care professionals. When she moved from Switzerland to the USA to live and work she was horrified by what she considered to be the appalling treatment of people who were dying. This led her to attack Western society as 'death-defying' (in Glaser and Strauss's terms, the whole of Western society was engaged in mutual pretence). What she and others who followed her approach argued was that dying and death should be much more accepted in the West as (the end) part of life, and that much could be learned from traditional societies about how best to handle the end of life. Moreover, Kubler-Ross through her work with people who were dying, believed that she had observed them going through a specific social process after they discovered that they had a terminal disease which was characterised by a series of emotional stages.

For Kubler-Ross, the first stage in this process is *denial*, whereby the patient refuses to believe that he/she is really going to die. Second, there is *anger*. At this stage the patient is resentful about dying, questioning why he/she has been singled out to die, and may become hostile towards those who are delivering care or relatives. The third stage is *bargaining*. Here the patient attempts to negotiate with those they consider have the power to reinterpret or reverse their advance towards death (for example, her/his medical practitioner, priest, or God). In the next stage, denial of, anger about, and bargaining over dying is replaced by a feeling of *depression*. Finally, there is *acceptance*, with the patient becoming calmer and readying himself/herself to let go of life and die peacefully.

Within this multi-staged psychological framework of dying, there is an assumption that the acceptance of death is more psychologically healthy for the patient than remaining in denial or continuing to execute rage. There is also a justification for the perpetration of open awareness. That is, it is assumed by Kubler-Ross that open awareness is an ethically correct approach and should be adopted by disease-care practitioners and relatives in their communications with the patient no matter which stage he/she has entered.

However, such a blanket policy of openness with regard to dying is culturally naive. Not only is there evidence that the stages of dying set out by Kubler-Ross cannot be generalised, but that no such scheme can possibly fit all the variants associated with human performance, nor the multitude of cultural differences that exist within the West (Young and Cullen, 1996).

Moreover, not addressing the complex effects of social structure and cultural diversity on individual performance is only part of the criticism that can be levelled at a policy of wholesale openness. By arguing that more notice should be taken of how other societies and cultures cope with dying and death, there is the assumption that the customs of the West are faulty. Hence Kubler-Ross and her followers are reproducing the essential paradox of the cultural relativist argument. There is an infeasible leap of logic from wanting to pay homage to the rightfulness of a number of (non-Western) cultures while criticising the 'wrongfulness' of other (Western) cultures. Put simply, what the correct conduct for a doctor, nurse, relative, and patient from New York, Edinburgh, or Melbourne should be in the dying process, cannot be extracted from observing what social scripts are followed when an Inuit, Fijian, or Peruvian Indian is dying. This is reverse cultural-imperialism. It is not the West that is (as is more usual) exporting its values to non-industrial or developing societies, but the values of the latter that are being imported to the West.

Indeed, it has been argued in a study by McIntosh (1977) that most of the patients he interviewed who were dying, although they knew they were extremely ill, did not want to know the actual diagnosis and prognosis for fear of discovering that they were going to die. Many of these patients, according to McIntosh, put forward questions and interpreted the information they were given in such a way as to have only good news about their condition. For disease-care practitioners to engender an open dialogue, therefore, would be both difficult and disrespectful of the patient's apparent wish to remain deluded. However, in McIntosh's study the patients' convoluted communications with medical staff were complicated further by the discrepancy between the overt and subliminal messages being given by doctors. Although the doctors stated that they would provide the patients with the facts regarding their illness, they were apparently reluctant to do so without a good deal of prompting.

Furthermore, Tony Walter (1991), examining the situation in Britain, argues that the notion of death being 'taboo' needs to be reassessed. He suggests that since the 1960s a more 'expressive' culture has developed, certainly among the middle classes, that makes death more possible to talk about. However, the reduction of death rates in modern society means that 'real' death does not occur as often, or when it does it happens out of sight within institutions. Moreover, most people who die today do so when they are elderly, rather than in the past when death was much more common among those in the prime of life. Previously, death was not only happening more frequently, but loss was experienced more intensely. The adults who died were important, if not essential, to the economy and emotional stability of their families. For Walter, therefore, it is hardly surprising that in the modern world people appear not to be competent at handling bereavement on a personal level, or that modern society does not possess meaningful ritualistic modes of expression in comparison with pre-modern societies. People today in the West are not 'denying' death. They have little opportunity to 'avow' death. Society, therefore, has barely any requirement for intricate and communal death liturgies. They may not even know the name of their neighbour who has died.

Moreover, as the world has become more and more influenced by Western values through globalisation, non-Western approaches to death and dying are more likely to become rarer. Global capitalism brings along its cultural attributes, some of which are noticeably moving the incidence of actual death from people's everyday experience into the experience of virtual death within cyberspace, and will probably establish a pattern of communication that doesn't sanctify openness as the norm.

A further study by Glaser and Strauss (1968) can also be considered a landmark in the re-conceptualisation of death and dying away from being understood merely as natural processes, and towards acknowledging their social significance. From their observations of dying in hospitals, Glaser and Strauss suggested that people who were dying went through various social phases, which they described as *Critical Junctures*. These junctures, which refer to the socially organised process of dying, are not to be confused with the psychological stages as denoted by Kubler-Ross. The difference is that Glaser and Strauss, rather than focusing mainly on the internal mechanisms of the dying person, were cognisant of the socio-environmental factors in the vicinity of a projected death and the effect of these factors on the patient's social status. For Glaser and Strauss, the patient who is dying undertakes a certain 'career pathway' from the point of the announcement of his/her terminal state to when death occurs. What should happen at each part of the dying career of the patient, and how long the career should last, is decreed by the expectations and reactions of the doctors and nurses who have responsibility for the patient, but who also have to take into account other administrative and organisational regulations and obligations. That is, the trajectory of the patient's dying career is mapped out by the doctors and nurses on the basis of what they believe to be the normal pattern for people with similar complaints. However, the bureaucratic design of the hospital will impinge on how the dying career of the patient is managed.

The ward staff may assume that a patient suffering from, for example, inoperable cancer of the stomach, with untreatable cancerous metastases in other organs, and who is irreversibly emaciated, will die within a few weeks. Local healthcare resources (which themselves are affected by health policies at a national level) will be formulated on the basis of how much care can be allocated to this patient, and similar patients. Staff shifts and numbers are arranged, and clinical equipment and palliative therapies ordered in an attempt to satisfy both the immediate needs of this patient and a generalised programme of care for others with equivalent diseases. Care is controlled, therefore, by financial considerations and organisational norms, as well as by clinical decisions.

There are commonly, suggest Glaser and Strauss, seven *Critical Junctures*. The first commences when the patient is defined as dying by the clinical staff. He/she is reclassified (perhaps unknowing if a *closed awareness* context is operating) from either a 'healthy person' or a 'patient' (i.e. a person with an illness) to a person who is 'dying'. Consequently, there is a dramatic loss of social standing as the label of 'dying' signifies a path towards being a person for whom there is no hope and no future. There is, therefore, a 'non-person' social ranking awaiting that individual as death approaches.

Michael Young and Lesley Cullen (1996) examined the meanings that fourteen patients, and their carers, attached to their lives following the diagnosis of cancer and having only a few months to live. Cancer, unlike, for example, death from a heart attack, represents a 'slow death'. Incidents of 'slow death' in the West are increasing, given the greater numbers of people dying from cancer compared to 'quick deaths' from infectious diseases, accidents, or wars. There is, therefore, with cancer a much greater chance of depersonalisation because dying is prolonged, but also because of the recognised severity of the disease:

> people quite suddenly stopped being people and became patients under someone else's orders. It was not for nothing that people customarily spoke of being 'under' – 'I am under the doctor' . . . They could cease overnight to be a person – or at any rate the same person when they were consigned to wait in giant buildings (the largest buildings many people go into) full of bustling strangers in white coats who, though strangers, may well have a terrifying power of clairvoyance about their future.
>
> (Young and Cullen, 1996: 38)

The second *Critical Juncture* happens when the relatives and friends of the dying person start to make emotional and practical preparations for the death. If the patient realises that he/she is going to die (particularly if there is an *Open Awareness* context), then he/she may also adjust emotionally to the situation. Following this, there will be, in the third *Critical Juncture*, what Glaser and Strauss describe as the 'nothing more to do' phase. That is, there has been a diagnosis and preparations for death have been made, but the individual concerned has not yet reached the steeply descending part of death career. There is, therefore, a lull in proceedings (practical and emotional) with loved ones not knowing how comforting they should be with the dying person. Medical and nursing staff may handle this period before the plunge towards death by avoiding close contact with the patient. It is at this point that the depersonalisation of the patient may become transparent.

The next four junctures involve overlapping phases which collectively make up the concluding interval of life. Lasting many hours or several days, the fourth *Critical Juncture* is classified as the 'final descent'. The routine on the hospital ward will alter noticeably. For example, the patient may be placed in a side-room and nursed more intensively. Extra pain-killing drugs or higher dosages may be prescribed. Visiting hours may be extended, with perhaps many more relatives and friends making an appearance. The fifth *Critical Juncture* heralds in the 'last hours' during which last rights may be administered or other religious ceremonies conducted. This is followed by the sixth *Critical Juncture*, the 'death watch'. Here a partner or near relative may choose to be with the dying person all day and night, or a nurse may be assigned to provide exclusive care and company.

Finally comes the death. Apart from being the catalyst for a number of cultural rituals depending on the dead person's faith (or lack of it), the death invokes all manner of organisational formalities: the medical sanctification of death; the reclassifying of the person from 'the patient' to 'the deceased'; the cleansing of the body; wrapping the body in a shroud; transfer of the body to the mortuary; the washing down of the (ex)patient's bed and removal of 'its' belongings; the registering of the event in the nurses' and doctors' records; informing the coroner.

So, the scene is preset for the patient to play his/her social role in the institutionalised drama of dying. All a dying patient has to do is to follow the designated trajectory towards death. This drama, however, is somewhat exceptional. Unlike most plays, the central character (and some of the supporting actors – that is, the relatives) have not been given a copy of the script. That is, the patient is generally unaware that a trajectory for her/his death has been formulated, and that her or his fate is being organised. Where the foreseen trajectory is not followed, and given the clandestine nature of its existence, it is highly possible that this will be a frequent occurrence, and there will be much consternation for both the relatives and the hospital staff. If, for example, the final descent is delayed (i.e. there is a slower trajectory than predicted) or sudden (i.e. there is a quicker trajectory than anticipated), then it may wreck the emotional strategies of the loved ones, and cause havoc to the administrative plans of the ward staff. Patients are expected,

DEATH

therefore, to die within their allotted trajectory 'with good grace' to have a 'good death'.

David Sudnow (1967), like Glaser and Strauss, has made a major contribution to the sociological study of death. His observations of the interactions between nursing and medical staff and their 'dead' patients in the emergency ward of a public hospital in the USA have illustrated how, depending on the condition and inferred social status of the patient, deaths are dealt with very differently. That is, there is a 'social inequality' in death and dying. Judgements are made by doctors and nurses about the prestige and character of a patient, with much more effort being made to revive those who are perceived to be young or wealthy, and much less effort delivered to those considered to be old or morally repugnant. The older a person is, the poorer she or he is considered to be, and the more socially undesirable, the quicker the pronouncement of death.

For example, Sudnow noticed that there was a dramatic eleven-hour long attempt by doctors and nurses to revive a young child who was brought into the emergency ward with the standard 'signs of death' (i.e. no detectable heart beat and the absence of breathing). However, the arrival of an elderly woman in the emergency ward with the same signs of death resulted in no medical intervention whatsoever, except that she was immediately pronounced dead.

In Sudnow's study, people who were regarded as alcoholics, 'dope' addicts, prostitutes, violent, vagrants, and those who had apparently committed suicide were generally declared dead relatively quickly. For Sudnow, however, any patient (dead or alive) who attends a public hospital in the USA is already denoted as socially 'inferior' compared to those who receive the services of private healthcare.

Akin to Glaser and Strauss's (1968) idea that dying people are depersonalised, Sudnow argued that a distinction can be drawn between 'biological' death and 'social' death. That is, Sudnow suggested that the hospital staff in his study regarded some patients who were not 'clinically' dead (i.e. the 'signs of life' – breathing and a palpable pulse – were still apparent) as corpses.

However, the reverse may also be true. Patients who die biologically (where there is a complete cessation of the body's organic functioning) may still be regarded as being 'alive' in that relatives may not accept that their loved one has died (Mulkay, 1993).

The biologically dead person may be talked to, or thought about, by his/her relatives as if the death had not occurred. Referring to the dead as though they are alive may either be short-lived (for example, the actuality of death may be affirmed by the attitude of hospital staff and the burial procedures), or long-term (for example, a lost child or partner may be considered to be surviving 'spiritually', embodied within an inanimate object).

Sudnow also commented on how people termed 'DOA' (dead on arrival) are dealt with. Ambulance staff were instructed to refer to people they suspected of being dead as 'possible' DOAs because only a physician could certify a 'sure' death. This procedure is demanded by the hospital authorities for legal and (in the USA) insurance purposes. Therefore, a person who is dead cannot be described as such until a doctor provides confirmation of that state. What, then, is the status of that person prior to the doctor's confirmation of death? Is she or he 'alive', or in an ontological void whereby she or he is neither living nor deceased?

In an update of Sudnow's work, Stefan Timmermans (1998) conducted a study of two USA hospitals in which he observed 112 scenes of resuscitation, and interviewed forty-two healthcare practitioners, including doctors, nurses, social workers, and chaplains. As Timmermans points out, the management of healthcare and medical science has changed dramatically since Sudnow's research in the 1960s. In particular, resuscitation theories, techniques, and equipment have been overhauled, and hospitals have installed formal 'protocols' indicating the correct procedures that should be followed by medical and nursing staff.

Paradoxically, argues Timmermans, these developments in medical science and the formalisation of practices have served merely to justify decisions made by hospital staff about who to resuscitate, and how much effort should be made to preserve life. Timmermans concludes that changes in healthcare practice have not altered substantially the appropriateness of Sudnow's concept of social inequalities in death. For example, age remains a major factor in determining the social viability of a patient. Moreover, if the disease-care workers involved in the resuscitation process identified the patient as a drunk or drug abuser, then less effort would be made. Aggressive use of the instruments of revival and implementation of medical protocols are preserved for those who are either known to those working in emergency wards, or who are perceived to have similar or higher cultural attributes. For the socially substandard, equipment and protocols are utilised ritualistically.

Timmermans' (2005, 2006) position is that the profession of medicine has sequestrated the right to ascribe culturally appropriate meanings to explain death throughout the West (and reinforces this social power to 'broker death' when its expertise is called upon to explicate suspicious or unobvious deaths). Globalisation, I suggest, will further expand medicine's power to broker death.

SUMMARY

Society is ambiguous towards death. Some deaths are encouraged blatantly. Huge numbers of people are killed in times of war. In times of peace, significant numbers of people are allowed to die as a consequence of how governments formulate and implement their policies, and the requirements of global capitalism. Moreover, while actual death is kept concealed, virtual death is flaunted. Death is a perpetual feature of news broadcasting and popular entertainment.

There is also ambiguity with respect to when a person can be classified as 'dying' and 'dead'. Both death and dying have become medical categories rather than natural events, and are affected by the contexts, junctures, and biases of the disease-care system. However, C. S. Lewis writing *A Grief Observed* about the death of his wife, Joy, displays no such ambiguity. His suffering is all too real:

> It is hard to have patience with people who say 'There is no death' or 'Death doesn't matter'. There is death . . . and it and they are irrevocable and irreversible. You might as well say that birth doesn't matter. I look up at the night sky. Is there anything more certain than that in all those vast times and spaces, if I were allowed to search for them, I should nowhere find her face, her voice, her touch? She dies. She is dead. Is the word so difficult to learn?
>
> (Lewis, 1961: 15)

After my neighbour's death, I did not feel the same degree of grief as Lewis at the loss of his wife. However, I am in accord with Lewis over the reality of death.

FURTHER READING

Howarth, G. (2006) *Death and Dying: A Sociological Introduction*. Cambridge: Polity Press.

MORAL ACTION

Explore (sensitively) the meaning of death with those who are dying or are grieving, and evaluate how you can alter/improve your interpersonal communications regarding death and dying and offer 'informed' support where appropriate (for example, the USA-based 'Citizens Against Homicide' publishes statements of those whose loved ones have been murdered, which I'm allowed to use for teaching purposes on the 'Madness and Murder' courses I run at the University of Leeds, and these have sensitised both me and my students to the impact of violence on people and society).

CONCLUSION

THERE IS NOT MEANT TO BE A CONCLUSION to this book. The writing and reading of it may be finished, but there is a moral obligation for the writer (me) and the reader (you) to continue with action.

The subjects covered in this book and the content delivered on those subjects is only an introduction to the sociology of health, and the problems of global disease and human suffering. Furthermore, the choice of subjects and content is biased by my experiences of learning and teaching the sociology of health, personal experiences of human suffering, and being jaded with the sociological elite and the lack of radicalism within or application of sociology to human suffering.

Throughout this book I have made the claim that we know that some things are real, but that there are other things we think are real but aren't as real as we think, and that there are yet other real things that we don't know about. Disease is real. Human suffering is real. I have also indicated that I have more admiration for people who attempt to tackle the reality of disease and suffering, such as Cecil Helman and Elizabeth Pisani, and remonstrated angrily against mental masturbation.

However, anger without action is the emotional equivalent of mental masturbation.

MORAL ACTION

William Easterly (2007) has argued that aid sent by the West to the underdeveloped world (particularly Africa) has been either squandered or pilfered, and in many instances has done more harm than good. Assessing where and how to take action is vital. Taking action should be judgement based on studying the problem and proposed resolutions by governments, agencies, and individuals. It may mean that you decide to organise a new response.

There are two levels that your and my action can embrace: practical and/or political.

1 Practical

The sociological imagination revealed in this book indicates how disease-care practitioners can make a difference to the immediate care of their patients. If you are a practitioner, then you should be aware of the problems associated in knowing what 'health' means to patients, how power operates within society, including the disease services, the dangers for patients from labelling and medicalisation, how flaky psychiatric diagnoses should not detract from the realisation that madness causes real mental pain, patients have sexual needs and that what is normal sexuality is mutating, human misery cannot be dismissed merely through pills and talk, and that death and dying matter to people, and require handling humanely not bureaucratically. You can be aware of these issues and act in accordance with that awareness. But most of all, doctors and nurses and other disciplines of disease, please be kind, competent, and clean.

2 Political

If you are a practitioner or a student from a non-practice-based discipline (and even an established academic), you can read about how to campaign for a better global society. For example, Bibi van der Zee's book *Rebel Rebel* (2007) provides guidelines about effective protesting. Duncan Green (2008) from Oxfam International offers insights into how 'active citizens' can empower themselves to effect change in their communities and globally, as well as arguing for better 'global governance' to reduce inequality and poverty. Requests can be made by you to your academic or professional organising bodies to take on a political dimension beyond that of representing its own interests. Remember, while your occupational body, trade union, or subject association is spending money on conferences at expensive hotels attempting to get better working conditions and salaries for its membership, or promote its power-base, children are dying in their millions.

Cecil Helman again:

Many children die young [in the underdeveloped world] – from infections, accidents, malnutrition, diarrhoeal diseases, many of them the diseases of poverty, made worse by poor education . . . I think . . . of the hundreds of hours I've spent over the years [in his London general practice] on sniffles and colds, minor blemishes and invisible rashes, all those lengthy talks only about trivia . . .

(Helman, 2006: 181)

POWER PENCILS

Finally, and perhaps wholly unrealistically for once, I concur with the intellectual and activist George Monbiot (2007a; 2008) who has evaluated many of the world's problems and concluded that the formation of global democratic government is necessary to solve them. A start would be for academics and practitioners to borrow a plea from Elizabeth Pisani (2008), to 'stand shoulder to shoulder against disease' and make a better global society. That is, the vanguard of a global government could be an alignment of the intelligentsia, doctors, nurses, physiotherapists, occupational therapists, psychotherapists, social workers, radiographers, audiologists, and every other discipline that cares to take action against global disease.

225

In any vanguard movement or global government that I get a chance to be part of I would ask to be in charge of nothing more than pencils – the distribution of pencils to those in global society who have no other means to write so that they can't be educated, and therefore cannot gain entry onto even the bottom rung of the social ladder, let alone enjoy one of the most valuable inventions of human civilisation, written communication. Being global pencil monitor would be a fitting career move and would save me from succumbing to the madness of mental masturbation.

REFERENCES

AfrOx (2008) 'Cancer in Africa'. Online at www.afrox.org.

Agence France-Presse (2008) 'EU ready to offer Iceland a loan, but it could take time: Reykjavik Nordic nations work on Iceland bail-out'. 7 November. Online at http://afp.google.com.

Allinson, T. (2007 [1893]) *Allinson's Essays*. Extracts edited by R. Metcalfe and K. MacDonald-Taylor. Peterborough: Allinson Flour.

American Association for the Advancement of Science – *Science* (2008) Medicine/Diseases (archived articles 1995–2008). Online at www.sciencemag.org/cgi/collection/medicine.

American College of Surgeons (2006) 'Unnecessary Operations'. Online at www.facs.org/fellows_info/statements/stonprin.html#anchor175181.

American Psychiatric Association (2000) *Diagnostic and Statistical Manual of Mental Disorders (DSM-IV-TR)*. Arlington, VA: American Psychiatric Association.

Andrews, J., Porter, R., Tucker, P. and Waddington, K. (1997) *The History of Bethlem*. London: Routledge.

Aries, P. (1983) *The Hour of Our Death*. Harmondsworth: Penguin.

Armstrong, D. (1984) 'The patient's view'. *Social Science and Medicine*, 18 (9): 737–744.

Associated Press (2006) 'Medical error "may have caused Sharon's stroke"'. *The Guardian*, 21 April.

Bacon, F. (1985 [1597]) '*Meditationes Sacræ. De Hæresibus*' [Religious Meditations, of Heresies]. In *The Essays*. Harmondsworth: Penguin.

Bakan, J. (2004) *The Corporation: The Pathological Pursuit of Profit and Power*. London: Constable & Robinson.

Baker, R. (1996) *Sperm Wars: Infidelity, Sexual Conflict, and Other Bedroom Battles*. London: Fourth Estate.

Barrett, J. (2004) 'Personal services or dangerous liaisons: should we help patients hire prostitutes?'. *British Medical Journal*, 329 (7472): 985.

Bataille, G. (1986 [1957]) *Eroticism, Death and Sexuality*. San Francisco, CA: City Lights.

Baudrillard, J. (1988) *Selected Writings*. Stanford, CA: Stanford University Press.

Baylis, N. (2005) *Learning from Wonderful Lives: Lessons from the Study of Well-being Brought to Life by the Personal Stories of Some Much Admired Individuals*. Cambridge: Cambridge Well-Being Books.

—— (2008) 'All about Nick's book and how to buy a copy'. Online at www.nickbaylis.com.

BBC Leeds (2007) 'Remembering Jane'. (Profiles.) Online at www.bbc.co.uk/leeds.

BBC News (2005) 'An acceptable career?'. 1 March. Online at http://news.bbc.co.uk.

—— (2008a) 'Firm "misled" over malaria drug. Cosmetics chain has dropped the sale of a homeopathic drug after watchdogs said customers were being misled that it could treat malaria'. 6 May. Online at http://news.bbc.co.uk.

—— (2008b) 'Baghdad bus stop bomb kills 51'. Online at http://news.bbc.co.uk/1/hi/world/middle_east/7459842.stm.

—— (2008c) 'Woman soldier among Afghan dead'. Online at http://news.bbc.co.uk.

Beck, U. (1992) *Risk Society: Towards A New Modernity* (trans.M. Ritter). London: Sage.

Becker, H. (1963) *Outsider: Studies in the Sociology of Deviance*. Glencoe: Free Press.

Bennett, C. (1998) 'In the blood or in the head?'. *The Guardian*, 1 June.

Ben-Shahar, T. (2007a) *Happier: Finding Pleasure, Meaning and Life's Ultimate Currency*. Maidenhead: McGraw-Hill.

—— (2007b) 'About Tal Ben-Shahar/Six happiness tips'. Online at http://talbenshahar.com.

—— (2008) 'Welcome to the positive psychology homepage'. Online at www.talbenshahar.com.

Benson, O. and Stangroom, J. (2006) *Why Truth Matters*. London: Continuum.

Bentall, R. (1992) 'A proposal to classify happiness as a psychiatric disorder'. *Journal of Medical Ethics*, 18 (20): 94–98.

—— (2003) *Madness Explained: Psychosis and Human Nature*. London: Allen Lane.

Berger, P. and Luckman, T. (1967) *The Social Construction of Reality: A Treatise in the Sociology of Knowledge*. Harmondsworth: Penguin.

Bhaskar, R. (2008) *A Realist Theory of Science*. London: Verso.

Blackburn, S. (2006) *Truth: A Guide for the Perplexed*. London: Penguin.

Blane, D. (1999) 'The life course, the social gradient, and health'. In M. Marmot and R. G. Wilkinson (eds) *Social Determinants of Health*. Oxford: Oxford University Press, pp. 64–80.

Blaxter, M. (1990) *Health and Lifestyles*. London: Tavistock.

Bocock, R. (1976) *Freud and Modern Society*. London: Van Nostrand Reinhold.

Bond, M. (2003) 'The pursuit of happiness'. *New Scientist*, 4 October, 180 (2415): 440–443.

Boseley, S. (1998) 'Medical studies "rubbish"'. *The Guardian*, 24 June.

—— (2006) 'Doctors urged [by British Medical Association] to be more vigilant over drugs' side-effects'. *The Guardian*, 12 May.

Boyle, M. (2002) *Schizophrenia: A Scientific Delusion* (2nd edn). London: Routledge.

Boyle, P., Gray, N., Henningfield, J., Seffrin, J. and Zatonski, W. (eds) (2004) *Tobacco: Science, Policy and Public Health*. Oxford: Oxford University Press.

Brown, L. R. (2008) *Plan B 3.0: Mobilizing to Save Civilization*. New York: Norton.

Brunelle, D. (2008) *From World Order to Global Disorder: States, Markets, and Dissent*. Vancouver, BC: University of British Columbia Press.

Burton, R. (2001 [1621]) *The Anatomy of Melancholy*. New York: New York Review Books.

—— (2004 [1621]) *The Anatomy of Melancholy: A Selection* (edited by K. Jackson). Manchester: Carcanet.

Busfield, J. (1986) *Managing Madness: Changing Ideas and Practice*. London: Unwin Hyman.

Buss, D. M. (1994) *The Evolution of Desire*. New York: Basic Books.

—— (2003) *Evolutionary Psychology: The New Science of the Mind*. Harlow: Allyn & Bacon.

Bywater, J. and Jones, R. (2007) *Sexuality and Social Work*. Exeter: Learning Matters.

Carvel, J. (2008) 'Minister's cure for "sicknote culture"'. *The Guardian*, 21 February.

Central Intelligence Agency (2008a) 'The World Factbook: Iceland'. Online at www.cia.gov/library/publications/the-world-factbook/geos/ic.html.

—— (2008b) 'The World Factbook: Bhutan'. Online at www.cia.gov/library/publications/the-world-factbook/geos/bt.html.

Chomsky, N. (2007) (2nd edn) *Hegemony or Survival: America's Quest for Global Dominance*. London: Penguin.

Cockerham, W. C. (2005) *Sociology of Mental Disorder* (7th edn). Upper Saddle River, NJ: Prentice Hall.

—— (2007) *Social Causes of Health and Disease*. Cambridge: Polity Press.

Cohen, S. and Taylor, L. (1992) *Escape Attempts: The Theory and Practice of Resistance to Everyday* (2nd edn). London: Routledge.

Collier, B. (2007) *The Bottom Billion: Why the Poorest Countries Are Failing and What Can Be Done About It*. Oxford: Oxford University Press.

Collins, B. E. and Raven, B. H. (1969) 'Group structure: attraction, coalitions, communication and power'. In G. Lindzey and E. Aronson (eds) *Handbook of Social Psychology* (Vol. 4, 2nd edn). Reading, MA: Addison-Wesley, pp. 102–204.

Commission on Growth and Development (2008) *The Growth Report: Strategies For Sustained Growth and Inclusive Development*. Washington, DC: Commission on Growth and Development.

Comte, A. (1853) *The Positive Philosophy* (trans. M. Martineau). London: Trubner.

Connell, R. W. (1996) *Masculinities*. Cambridge: Polity Press.

Conrad, P. and Schneider, J. (1980) *Deviance and Medicalisation: From Badness to Sickness*. St. Louis, MI: Mosby.

Coppock, V. and Hopton, J. (2000) *Critical Perspectives on Mental Health*. London: Routledge.

Crawford, R. (1980) 'Healthism and the medicalisation of everyday life'. *International Journal of Health Services*, 10: 365–88.

Danner, D., Snowdon, D. and Friesen, W. (2001) 'Positive emotions in early life and longevity: findings from the nun study'. *Journal of Personality and Social Psychology*, 80: 804–813.

Darwin, C. (1998 [1859]) *The Origin of Species*. Oxford: Oxford World's Classics.

Davey, B. and Seale, C. (1996) (eds) *Experiencing and Explaining Disease*. Buckingham: Open University Press.

Davey-Smith, G. (2003) *Health Inequalities: Life Course Approaches*. Bristol: Policy Press.

Dawkins, R. (1994) 'Science's social standing: the moon is not a calabash'. *The Times Higher Education Supplement*, 30 September.

—— (1997) 'Is science a religion?' *The Humanist*, January/February, 57 (1). Online at www.thehumanist.org.

—— (2006) *The God Delusion*. London: Bantam Press.

de Bernières, L. (1994) *Captain Corelli's Mandolin*. London: Vintage.

Delanty, G. (1997) *Social Science: Beyond Constructivism and Realism*. Buckingham: Open University Press.

Dellar, R., Curtis, T. and Leslie, E. (eds) (2000) *Mad Pride*. London: Chipmunkapublishing.

Descartes, R. (2007 [1637]) *Discourse on Method and the Meditations*. London: Penguin.

Dey, I. (2008) 'Is Iceland headed for meltdown?' *Daily Telegraph*, 15 February. Online at www.telegraph.co.uk.

Diagnostic Clinic (2005) 'Almost 70% of people say complementary medicine is as valid as conventional'. Press release, 24 January. London: Diagnostic Clinic.

Diamond, J. (2001) 'Snake oil folklore, hocus pocus, mysticisms, and purveyors of snake oil'. In Dominic Lawson (ed.) *Snake Oil and Other Preoccupations* (Foreword by Richard Dawkins). London: Vintage.

Diener, R. (2001) 'Making the best of a bad situation: satisfaction in the slums of Calcutta'. *Social Indicators Research*, 55: 329–352.

Drysdale, G. (1861) *The Elements of Social Science: Or Physical, Sexual, and Natural Religion* (4th edn). London: Truelove.

Dunn, E., Aknin, L. and Norton, M. (2008) 'Spending money on others promotes happiness'. *Science*, 319 (5870): 1687–1688.

Durkheim, E, (1966 [1897]) *Suicide*. New York: Free Press.

Eady, J. (2008) Full judgement in case number HQO801303X, *Max Mosely vs. News Group Newspapers Limited*, 24 July. London: The Royal Courts of Justice.

Easterbrook, G. (2004) *The Progress Paradox: How Life Gets Better While People Feel Worse*. New York: Random House.

Easterly, W. R. (2007) *The White Man's Burden: Why the West's Efforts to Aid the Rest Have Done So Much Ill and So Little Good*. Oxford: Oxford University Press.

Economic and Social Research Council (2008) *Global Life Expectancy 2008*. London: ESRC.

Economist Editorial (2006) 'Happiness and economics: economics discovers its feelings'. *The Economist*, 19 December.

Edwards, N. (2008) 'Talking about a revolution, but which one?' *The Guardian*, 18 June.

Einsiedel, E. (2008) (ed.) *Public Understanding of Science*. Thousand Oaks, CA: Sage.

Elliott, A. and Lemert, C. (2005) *The New Individualism: The Emotional Costs of Globalization*. London: Routledge.

Elliot, L. and Atkinson, D. (2008) *The Gods that Failed. How Blind Faith in Markets Has Cost Us our Future*. London: Bodley Head.

Emmel, N. D. and D'Souza, L. (1999) 'Health effects of forced evictions in the slums of Mumbai'. *The Lancet*, 25 September, 354: 1118.

Engels, F. (1845) *The Condition of the Working Class in England [Die Lage der arbeitenden Klasse in England]*. Leipzig: Frow.

——— (1999 [1892]) *The Condition of the Working Class in England*. Oxford: Oxford Paperbacks.

English Collective of Prostitutes (2006) 'Report to the UN Special Rapporteur on Violence Against Women'. London: English Collective of Prostitutes.

Esty, A. (2004) 'The new wealth of nations: does Bhutan have a better way to measure national progress?' *American Scientist*, 92 (6), November-December. Online at www.americanscientist.org.

Evans, M. (2005) *Killing Thinking: The Death of the Universities* (2nd edn). New York: Continuum.

Evans-Pritchard, E. E. (1937) *Witchcraft, Oracles and Magic Among the Azande*. Oxford: Clarendon.

Families USA (2007) *Wrong Direction: One Out of Three Americans Are Uninsured*. USA: Families USA.

Faris, R. and Dunham, W. (1965). *Mental Disorders in Urban Areas*. Chicago, IL: University of Chicago Press.

Fennell, P. (1996) *Treatment Without Consent: Law, Psychiatry and the Treatment of Mentally Disordered People Since 1845*. London: Routledge.

Ferrie, J. E. (ed.) (2004) *Work Stress and Health: The Whitehall II Study*. London: International Centre for Health and Society/Department of Epidemiology and Public Health, University College.

Feyerabend, P. (1975) *Against Method*. London: New Left Books.

Field, D. (1989) *Nursing the Dying*. London: Tavistock/Routledge.

Financial Times (2008) 'Global financial crisis'. Online at www.ft.com/indepth/global-financial-crisis.

Fitzpatrick, M. (2000) *The Tyranny of Health: Doctors and the Regulation of Lifestyle*. London: Routledge.

Fletcher, N. (2008) 'Hyperactivity drug goes too slow for Shire'. *The Guardian*, 7 May.

Forbes (2008) 'The world's billionaires'. Online at www.forbes.com/billionaires.

Forrester, V. (1999) *The Economic Horror*. Cambridge: Polity Press.

Foucault, M. (1961) *Histoire de la folie à l'âge classique* (translated as *Madness and Civilization*). Paris: Plon.

—— (1969) *Archaeology of Knowledge* [*L'Archéologie du Savoir*]. London: Routledge.

—— (1973) *The Birth of the Clinic: An Archaeology of Medical Perception*. New York: Pantheon.

—— (1975) *Surveiller et punir: Naissance de la prison*. Paris: Gallimard.

—— (1980) *Power/Knowledge, Selected Interviews and Other Writings 1972–1977*. Brighton: Harvester.

—— (1985) *The History of Sexuality: The Use of Pleasure* (Vol. 2). Harmondsworth: Penguin.

Freidson, E. (1970) *The Profession of Medicine: A Study of the Applied Sociology of Knowledge*. New York: Dodd Mead.

—— (1971) *Professional Dominance: The Social Structure of Medical Care*. Chicago, IL: Aldine.

—— (1988) *Professional Powers: A Study of the Institutionalization of Formal Knowledge*. Chicago, IL: University of Chicago Press.

—— (1994) *Professionalism Reborn: Theory, Prophecy and Policy*. Cambridge: Polity Press.

—— (2001) *Professionalism, the Third Logic: On the Practice of Knowledge*. Chicago, IL: University of Chicago Press.

French, H. (2006) 'Chinese paradise is hell for most low-level workers'. *International Herald Tribune* (*New York Times*), 18 December.

French, J. R. P. and Raven, B. H. (1959) 'The bases of social power'. In D. Cartwright (ed.) *Studies in Social Power*. Michigan, MI: University of Michigan Press, pp. 150–167.

Freud, S. (1930) 'Civilisation and its discontents'. In J. Strachey (ed.) *The Standard Edition of the Complete Works of Sigmund Freud* (Volume XXI). London: Hogarth.

Friday, N. (1976) *My Secret Garden: Women's Sexual Fantasies*. London: Quartet Books.

—— (1991) *Women on Top: How Real Life Has Changed Women's Sexual Fantasies*. London: Hutchinson.

Fromm, E. (1963) *The Sane Society*. London: Routledge & Kegan Paul.

Fugh-Berman, A. (2005) 'Not in my name: how I was asked to "author" a ghost-written research paper'. *The Guardian*, 21 April.

Fuller, S. (2007a) *New Frontiers in Science and Technology Studies*. Cambridge: Polity Press.

—— (2007b) *The Knowledge Book: Key Concepts in Philosophy, Science and Culture*. Stocksfield, Northumberland: Acumen.

Furedi, F. (2003) *Therapy Culture*. London: Routledge

—— (2004) *Where Have All the Intellectuals Gone?: Confronting 21st Century Philistinism*. London: Continuum.

Gates, B. (2000) 'Shaping the internet age'. Online at www.microsoft.com.

Geary, R. (1998) *Essential Criminal Law* (2nd edn). London: Cavendish.

Geddes, L. (2008) 'Ultrasound nails location of the elusive G spot'. *New Scientist*, 20 February, 2644: 6–7.

Giddens, A. (1991) *Modernity and Self-identity: Self and Society in the Late Modern Age*. Cambridge: Polity Press.

—— (2006) *Sociology* (5th edn). Cambridge: Polity Press.

Giridharadas, A. (2006) 'Not everyone is grateful as investors build free apartments in Mumbai slums'. *New York Times*, 15 December.

Glaser, B. and Strauss, A. (1965) *Awareness of Dying*. Chicago, IL: Aldine.

—— and —— (1968) *Time For Dying*. Chicago, IL: Aldine.

Global Fund (2008) 'The Global Fund, an NGO set-up to fight AIDS, tuberculosis and malaria'. Online at www.theglobalfund.org/EN/aria.

Glyn, A. (2006) *Capitalism Unleashed: Finance, Globalization, and Welfare*. Oxford: Oxford University Press.

Goffman, E. (1959) *The Presentation of Self in Everyday Life*. New York: Doubleday.

—— (1961) *Asylums: Essays on the Social Situation of Mental Patients and Other Inmates*. New York: Doubleday.

—— (1963) *Stigma: Notes on the Management of Spoiled Identity*. Upper Saddle River, NJ: Prentice-Hall.

Goldacre, B. (2008a) *Bad Science*. London: Fourth Estate.

—— (2008b) 'It's not just about Prozac. Our failure to properly regulate testing in the pharmaceutical industry has devastating costs'. *The Guardian*, 27 February.

—— (2008c) 'Pixie dust helps man grow new finger'. *Bad Science*. Online at www.badscience.net.

Goodwin, B. (2007) *Nature's Due: Healing Our Fragmented Culture*. Edinburgh: Floris.

Goodwin, S. (1997) *Comparative Mental Health Policy*. London: Sage.

Gramsci, A. (1971) *Selections from the Prison Notebooks* (trans. and eds, Q. Hoare and G. N. Smith). New York: International Publishers.

Greaves, D. (2000) 'The quality of life: the obsessive pursuit of health and happiness'. *British Medical Journal*, 321 (7276): 1572–1576.

Green, C. (2004) *The Little Book of Loony Sex Laws*. Glasgow: VitalSpark.

Green, D. (2008) *From Poverty to Power*. Oxford: Oxfam International.

Greenhalgh, T. and Wessely, S. (2004) '"Health for me": A sociocultural analysis of healthism in the middle classes'. *British Medical Bulletin*, 69: 197–213.

Greenpeace (2006) 'Eating up the Amazon'. 6 April. Online at www.greenpeace.org/raw/content/international/press/reports/eating-up-the-amazon.pdf.

Greer, G. (1970) *The Female Eunuch*. London: MacGibbon & Kee.

Gribbin, J. (2003) *Science: A History 1534–2001*. London: Penguin.

Guardian Soulmates (2008) 'Dating'. Online at www.guardian.co.uk.

Halliday, S. (2007) *The Great Filth: The War Against Disease in Victorian England*. London: Sutton.

Hammond, C. (2008) 'Africa's looming cancer epidemic'. *BBC News*, 12 June. Online at http://news.bbc.co.uk.

Hart, G. and Wellings, K. (2002) 'Sexual behaviour and its medicalisation: in sickness and in health', *British Medical Journal*, 13 April, 324: 896–900.

Hawkes, G. (1996) *A Sociology of Sex and Sexuality*. Buckingham: Open University Press.

Hobbes, T. (1998 [1651]) *Leviathan*. Oxford: Oxford University Press.

Haynes, B., Devereaux, P. and Guyatt, G. (2002) 'Physicians' and patients' choices in evidence based practice: evidence does not make decisions, people do'. *British Medical Journal*, 8 June, 324 (7350): 1350.

Hazelton, M. and Morrall, P. (2008) 'Mental health, the law, and human rights'. In P. Barker (ed.) *Psychiatric and Mental Health Nursing: The Craft of Caring*. London: Hodder Arnold, Chapter 70.

Healthcare Commission (2008) 'National survey of NHS staff 2007'. London: Commission for Healthcare Audit and Inspection.

Health Protection Agency (2008) 'More antibiotic development needed warns Health Protection Agency'. Press release, 10 September. Online at www. hpa.org.uk.

Helman, C. (2006) *Suburban Shaman: Tales from Medicine's Frontline*. London: Hammersmith Press.

—— (2007) *Culture, Health and Illness* (5th edn). London: Hodder Arnold.

Hirsch, I. B. (2002) 'Unproven therapies'. *Clinical Diabetes*, 20: 1–3.

Hitchens, C. (2007) *God Is Not Great: The Case Against Religion*. London: Atlantic Books.

Holmes, B., Kleiner, K., Douglas, K. and Bond, M. (2003) 'Reasons to be cheerful'. *New Scientist*, 4 October, 2415.

Hopkirk, E. (2005) 'Blunders by doctors killed runner'. *Evening Standard*, 28 February.

Hughes, J. (1991) *An Outline of Modern Psychiatry* (3rd edn). Chichester: Wiley.

Illich, I. (1975) *Medical Nemesis: The Expropriation of Health*. London: Marian Boyars.

——, Zola, I. and McKnight, J. (1977) *Disabling Professions*. London: Marion Boyars, Chapter 1, pp. 11–39.

James, O. (2007) *Affluenza*. London: Vermilion.

—— (2008) *The Selfish Capitalist*. London: Vermilion.

Jha, A. (2007) 'From arthritis to diabetes: scientists unlock genetic secrets of diseases afflicting millions'. *The Guardian*, 7 June.

—— (2008) 'Scientists hail spinal injury breakthrough. Researchers use bypass technique to restore movement in paralysed rats'. *The Guardian*, 7 February.

——, Jacob, B., Gajalakshmi, V., Gupta, P., Dhingra, N., Kumar, R., Sinha, D., Dikshit, R. Parida, D., Kamadod, R., Boreham, J. and Peto, R. (2008) 'A nationally representative case-control study of smoking and death in India'. *New England Journal of Medicine*, 358 (11): 1137–1147.

Joannides, P. and Gross, D. (1999) *The Guide To Getting It On!* West Hollywood, CA: Goofy Foot Press. Online at http://boinkcentral.com/menu.html.

Johnstone, L. (2000) *Users and Abusers of Psychiatry. A Critical Look at Psychiatric Practice* (2nd edn). London: Brunner-Routledge.

Jones, K., Patelm N., Levy, M., Storeygard, A., Balk, D., Gittleman, J. and Daszak, P. (2008) 'Global trends in emerging infectious diseases'. *Nature* 451: 990–993.

Kellehear, A. (2007) *A Social History of Dying*. Cambridge: Cambridge University Press.

Kilvert, F. (1978) *Kilvert's Diary: Selections From the Diary of the Reverend Francis Kilvert 1870–1879* (W. Plomer, ed.). London: Book Club Associates.

Kinsey, A., Pomeroy, W. and Martin, C. (1948) *Sexual Behavior in the Human Male*. Philadelphia, PA: Saunders.

——, —— and —— (1953) *Sexual Behavior in the Human Female*. Philadelphia, PA: Saunders.

Kirby, J. (2008) 'Obituary Keith Ball: cardiologist, medical campaigner and co-founder of Ash'. *The Guardian*, 11 February.

Kirsch, I., Deacon, B., Huedo-Medina, T., Scoboria, A., Moore, T. and Johnson, B. (2008) 'Initial severity and antidepressant benefits: a meta-analysis of data submitted to the food and drug administration'. *Public Library of Science Journal*. Online at http://medicine.plosjournals.org.

Klein, N. (2007) *The Shock Doctrine: The Rise of Disaster Capitalism*. London: Allen Lane.

Kramer, P. (1993) *Listening to Prozac: The Landmark Book About Antidepressants and the Remaking of the Self*. New York: Penguin.

—— (1994) *Listening to Prozac: A Psychiatrist Explores Antidepressant Drugs and Remaking of the Self*. London: Fourth Estate.

Kubler-Ross, E. (1969) *On Death and Dying*. New York: Macmillan.

Kuhn, T. (1962) *The Structure of Scientific Revolutions*. Chicago, IL: University of Chicago Press.

Laing, R. D. (1960*)* *The Divided Self: An Existential Study in Sanity and Madness*. Harmondsworth: Penguin.

—— and Esterson, A. (1964) *Sanity, Madness and the Family*. Harmondsworth: Penguin.

Layard, R. (2006) *Happiness: Lessons from a New Science*. Harmondsworth: Penguin.

Leader, D. (2007) 'A dark age for mental health – a therapy last used on a mass scale in China's cultural revolution is to be unleashed on the NHS'. *The Guardian*, 13 October.

—— (2008) 'The creation of the Prozac myth'. *The Guardian*, 27 February.

Legrain, P. (2003) *Open World: The Truth About Globalisation*. London: Abacus.

Lemert, E. (1951) *Social Pathology: A Systematic Approach to the Study of Sociopathic Behavior*. New York: McGraw-Hill.

Lewis, A. (1953) 'Health as a social concept'. *British Journal of Sociology*, 2 (4): 109–124.

Lewis, C. S. (1961*) A Grief Observed*. London: Faber & Faber

Lindberg, C. (1992) *The Beginnings of Western Science: The European Scientific Tradition in Philosophical, Religious, and Institutional Context, 600 BC to AD 1450*. Chicago, IL: University of Chicago Press.

Lovelock, J. (2007*) The Revenge of Gaia: Why the Earth Is Fighting Back and How We Can Still Save Humanity*. London: Penguin.

Lukes, S. (1974) *Power: A Radical View*. London: Macmillan.

McGreal, C. (2008a) 'George Bush: a good man in Africa: as he starts a five-nation tour, the US president is an unlikely hero to the poor of a continent ravaged by AIDS'. *The Guardian*, 15 February.

—— (2008b) 'Nigeria takes on big tobacco over campaigns that target the young'. *The Guardian*, 15 January.

McIntosh, J. (1977) *Communication and Awareness in a Cancer Ward*. London: Croom Helm.

McKeown, T. (1976) *The Role of Medicine: Dream, Mirage, or Nemesis?* London: Nuffield Provincial Hospitals Trust.

McKie, R. (2005) 'Professor savages homeopathy'. *The Observer*, 18 December.

McQuail, D. (2005) *McQuail's Mass Communication Theory* (5th edn). London: Sage.

McVeigh, T. (2008) 'The party's over for Iceland, the island that tried to buy the world'. *The Observer*, 5 October.

Maguire, K. and Campbell, D. (2000) 'Tobacco giant implicated in global smuggling schemes'. *The Guardian*, 31 January.

Make Roads Safe (2008) 'The issues (Campaign for Global Road Safety)'. Online at www.makeroadssafe.org/issues/index/html.

Marmot, M. (2008) 'Commission on social determinants of health – what is our focus? World Health Organization'. Online at www.who.int/social_determinants/advocacy/interview_marmot/en.

—— , Shipley, M. J. and Rose, G. (1984) 'Inequalities in death – specific explanations of a general pattern?'. *Lancet*, 5 May, 1: 1003–1006.

Marshall, T. (2000) 'Exploring fiscal food policy: the case of diet and ischaemic heart disease'. *British Medical Journal*, 320: 301–305.

Marx, K. (1959 [1844]) *Economic and Philosophical Manuscripts of 1844* (ed. D. Struik; trans. M. Milligan). London: Lawrence & Wishart.

—— (1971 [1867]) *Das Kapital/Capital: A Critique of Political Economy* (ed. F. Engels). London: Lawrence & Wishart.

Match.Com (2008) Online at http://uk.match.com/help/aboutus.aspx.

Mathews, R. (1998) 'Flukes and flaws'. *Prospect*, November: 20–24.

Mechanic, D. (1968) *Medical Sociology*. New York: Free Press.

—— (2003) 'Who shall lead: Is there a future for population health?'. *Journal of Health Politics, Policy and Law*, 28 (2–3): 2421–2442.

Merton, R. K. (1938) 'Social structure and anomie'. *American Sociological Review*, 3 (October): 672–682.

Miah, A. and Rich, E. (2006) *The Medicalisation of Cyberspace*. London: Routledge.

Mill, J. S. (2001 [1861]) *Utilitarianism* (ed. G. Sher; 2nd edn). Indianapolis, Indiana, IN: Hackett.

Miller, J. (1993) *The Passion of Michel Foucault*. New York: Simon & Schuster.

Miller, P. and Rose, N. (1986) *The Power of Psychiatry*. Cambridge: Polity Press.

Millett, K. (1977) *Sexual Politics*. London: Virago.

236

Mills, C. W. (1959) *The Sociological Imagination*. Oxford: Oxford University Press.

Monbiot, G. (2007a) *The Age of Consent: A Manifesto for a New World Order*. London: Blackwell.

—— (2007b) *Heat: How We Can Stop the Planet Burning*. London: Penguin.

—— (2008) 'Globalising.org'. Online at www.globalising.org.

Monty Python (1983) *The Meaning of Life* [film]. Hollywood, LA: Universal Pictures.

Morris, C. (2008) 'Bhutan experiments with democracy'. *BBC News*, 25 March. Online at http://news.bbc.co.uk.

Morrall, P. A. (1998) *Mental Health Nursing and Social Control*. London: Whurr.

—— (2000) *Madness & Murder*. London: Whurr.

—— (2001) *Sociology and Nursing*. London: Routledge.

—— (2006a) *Murder and Society*. Chichester: Wiley.

—— (2006b) 'Psychiatry and psychiatric nursing in the new world order'. In J. Cutcliffe and M. Ward (eds) *Key Debates in Psychiatric/Mental Health Nursing*. Oxford: Elsevier.

—— (2008a) 'Snake Oil peddling: complementary and alternative medicine and the occupational status of doctors and nurses'. In J. Adams and P. Tovey (eds) *Complementary and Alternative Medicine in Nursing and Midwifery: Towards a Critical Social Science*. London: Routledge, pp. 52–69.

—— (2008b) *The Trouble With Therapy*. Maidenhead: Open University Press/ McGraw-Hill.

—— (2009) 'Provocation: reviving thinking in universities'. In T. Warne and S. McAndrew (eds) *Creative Approaches in Health and Social Care Education and Practice: Knowing Me, Understanding You*. London: Palgrave.

—— and Hazelton, M. (2004) *Mental Health: Global Policies and Human Rights*. Chichester: Wiley.

Morris, S. (2008) 'Pay-per-view service at crematorium'. *The Guardian*, 31 March.

Mulkay, M. (1993) 'Death in Britain'. In D. Clark (ed.) *The Sociology of Death*. Oxford: Blackwell, Chapter 2, pp. 31–49.

Museo Larco (2007) 'Aztec eroticism in ceramics: Lima, Peru: Museo Larco'. Online at http://museolarco.perucultural.org.pe/iindex.html.

Nassim, Taleb (2006) *The Black Swan: The Impact of the Highly Improbable*. London: Palgrave Macmillan.

Nestle, M. (2007) *Food Politics: How the Food Industry Influences Nutrition and Health* (2nd edn). Berkeley, CA: University of California Press.

Nettleton, S. (2004) 'The emergence of e-scaped medicine?' *Sociology*, 38 (4): 661–679.

Nettleton, S. (2006) *The Sociology of Health and Illness* (2nd edn). Cambridge: Polity Press.

New Internationalist (unattributed) (2008) 'For the happiness of individuals: sex rights – Poland and Latvia'. January, p. 12.

Oral Cancer Foundation (2008) 'The last taboo'. Online at www.oralcancer foundation.org.

237

Oxfam (2008) *Oxfam International Position on Food Prices*. Oxford: Oxfam International.

Parker, G. (2007) 'Is depression overdiagnosed?' *British Medical Journal*, 335 (7615): 328.

Parsons, T. (1951) *The Social System*. New York: Free Press of Glencoe.

Patterson, R. and Weijer, C. (1998) 'D'oh! An analysis of the medical care provided to the family of Homer J. Simpson'. *Canadian Medical Association Journal*, 15 December, 159 (12): 1480–1481.

Pearce, F. (2006) *The Last Generation*. Bodelva, St Austell: Eden Project Books.

Perrons, D. (2004) *Globalisation and Social Change: People and Places in a Divided World*. London: Routledge.

Picard, L. (2006) *Victorian London: The Life of a City 1840–1870*. London: Orion.

Pilkington, E. (2007) 'Insurer's U-turn too late to save life of transplant teenager. Lawyer wants company to be charged with murder: death inflames debate over US healthcare system'. *The Guardian*, 22 December.

Pisani, E. (2008) *The Wisdom of Whores: Bureaucrats, Brothels and the Business of AIDS*. London: Granta.

Pope, W. (1976) *Durkheim's 'Suicide': A Classic Analyzed*. Chicago, IL: University of Chicago.

Popper, K. (1959) *The Logic of Scientific Discovery*. New York: Harper & Row.

Porter, R. (1987) *A Social History of Madness: Stories of the Insane*. London: Weidenfeld & Nicolson.

—— (2002) *Blood and Guts: A Short History of Medicine*. London: Penguin.

—— (2003) *Madness: A Brief History*. Oxford: Oxford University Press.

Public Library of Science – Medicine (2006) Online at http://medicine.plos journals.org.

Putnam, R. (2006) (quoted by M. Easton, home editor, BBC News) 'The happiness formula – does happiness live in cyberspace?'. Online at http://news. bbc.co.uk/1/hi/programmes/happiness_formula/5052078.stm (accessed 7 June).

Radley, A. (1994) *Making Sense of Illness: The Social Pathology of Health and Disease*. London: Sage.

Redelmeier, D. and Kahneman, D. (1996) 'Patients' memories of painful medical treatments: real time and retrospective evaluations of two minimally invasive procedures'. *Pain*, July, 66 (1): 3–8.

—— , Katz, J. and Kahneman, D. (2003) 'Memories of colonoscopy: a randomized trial'. *Pain*, July, 104 (1–2): 187–94.

Reeves, S., Nelson, S. and Zwarenstein, M. (2008) 'The doctor–nurse game in the age of interprofessional care: a view from Canada'. *Nursing Inquiry*, 15 (1): 1–2.

Richman, J. (1987) *Medicine and Health*. London: Longman.

Roehr, B. (2006) 'Institute of Medicine report strives to reduce medication errors'. *British Medical Journal*, 29 July, 333: 220.

Robertson, A., Brunner, E. and Sheilam, A. (1999) 'Food is a political issue'. In M. Marmot and R. G. Wilkinson (eds) *Social Determinants of Health*. Oxford: Oxford University Press, Chapter 9, pp. 179–208.

Rogers, A. and Pilgrim, D. (2005) *A Sociology of Mental Health and Illness* (3rd edn). Maidenhead: Open University Press.

Rogers, C. (1951) *Client Centred Therapy*. London: Constable.

Rose, N. (2000) 'Government and control'. *British Journal of Criminology*, 40 (2): 321–339.

Rose, S. (1997) *Lifelines: Biology, Freedom, Determinism*. Harmondsworth: Penguin.

Rosen, D. (2006) 'Imperialism's second front: Bush's foreign sex policy'. *Counterpunch*, 22 December. Online at www.counterpunch.org/rosen1222 2006.html.

Russell, B. (1961) *History of Western Civilisation*. London: Routledge.

Scheerer, S. and Hess, H. (1997) 'Social control: a defence and reformulation. In R. Bergalli and C. Sumner (eds) *Social Control and Political Order: European Perspectives at the End of the Century*. London: Sage, Chapter 5, pp. 96–130.

Scheff, T. J. (1966) *Being Mentally Ill: A Sociological Theory*. Chicago, IL: Aldine.

Schumaker, J. F. (2006) 'The happiness conspiracy: what does it mean to be happy in a modern consumer society?' *New Internationalist*, July, Issue 391. Online at www.newint.org/columns/essays/2006/07/01/happinessconspiracy.

Scull, A. T. (1984) *Decarceration: Community Treatment and the Deviant – A Radical View* (2nd edn). Cambridge: Polity Press.

Scull, A. (1992) *Social Order – Mental Disorder: Anglo-American Psychiatry in Historical Perspective*. Berkeley, CA: University of California Press.

—— (2007) 'The fictions of Foucault's scholarship'. *The Times Online*. Online at http://tls.timesonline.co.uk.

Sebrié, E. and Glantz, S. (2006) 'The tobacco industry in developing countries'. *British Medical Journal*, 11 February, 332: 313–314.

Seligman, M. (2008) 'Authentic happiness'. Online at www.authentichappiness. sas.upenn.edu.

Sense About Science (2007) 'Malaria & homeopathy'. Online at www.sense aboutscience.org.uk.

Shilling, C. (2007) 'Sociology and the body: classical traditions and new agendas'. *Sociological Review* 55 (1): 1–18.

Shiva, V. (2000) BBC Reith Lecture 2000 'Poverty and globalisation'. Online at http://news.bbc.co.uk/hi/english/static/events/reith_2000/lecture5.stm.

Shoffman, M. (2006) 'Entertainers outraged by another gay murder'. 27 September. Online at www.pinknews.co.uk.

Shorter, E. (1997) *A History of Psychiatry*. Wiley: New York.

Singer, P. (1975) *Animal Liberation*. New York: Ecco Books.

—— (1995) *Rethinking Life and Death*. New York: St Martin's Griffin.

—— (2004) *One World: The Ethics of Globalization*. New Haven, CT: Yale University Press.

Singh, S. and Ernst, E. (2008) *Trick or Treatment?: Alternative Medicine on Trial*. London: Bantam Press.

Smallwood, C. (2005) *The Role of Complementary and Alternative Therapy in the NHS*. London: Freshminds Consultancy.

239

Smith, R. (2002) 'In Search of "Non-Disease"'. *British Medical Journal*, 13 April, 324: 883–885.

—— and Moynihan, R. (2002) 'Too much medicine? Almost certainly'. *British Medical Journal*, 13 April, 324: 859–860.

Social Trends (2008). 'Wealthier and healthier but are we happier?'. Press release, Social Trends, 38th edn. London: Office for National Statistics.

Sokal, A. and Bricmont, J. (2003) *Intellectual Impostures* (2nd edn). London: Economist Books.

Sontag, S. (1990) *Illness as Metaphor/AIDS and its Metaphors*. New York: Doubleday.

Stein, L. (1967) 'The doctor–nurse game'. *Archives of General Psychiatry*, 12: 699–703.

Stone, M. (1998) *Healing the Mind: A History of Psychiatry from Antiquity to the Present*. London: Pimlico.

Sudnow, D. (1967) *Passing On: The Social Organisation of Dying*. New York: Prentice Hall.

Szasz, T. S. (1972) *The Myth of Mental Illness*. St Albans: Paladin.

—— (1993) 'Curing, coercing, and claims-making: a reply to critics'. *British Journal of Psychiatry*, 162: 797–800.

—— (1994) 'Mental illness is still a myth'. *Society*, 31 (4): 34–39.

—— (1998) 'Parity for mental illness, disparity for the mental patient'. *Lancet*, 352 (9135): 1213–1215.

—— and Hollender, M. H. (1956) 'A contribution to the philosophy of medicine'. *American Medical Association's Archives of Internal Medicine*, XCVII, 585592.

Taleb, N. (2006) *The Black Swan: The Impact of the Highly Improbable*. London: Palgrave Macmillan.

Tallis, R. (2004) *Hippocratic Oaths: Medicine and its Discontents*. London: Atlantic.

Tannen, D. (1992) *You Just Don't Understand: Women and Men in Conversation*. London: Virago.

Templar, R. (2005) *The Rules of Life: A Personal Code for Living a Better, Happier, More Successful Kind of Life*. London: Pearson.

Thagard, P. (2005) *Mind: Introduction to Cognitive Science* (2nd edn). Cambridge, MA: MIT Press.

The Fat Task Force (2008) 'About the FATF'. Online at www.naafa.org/fatf.

The Laser Vagina Rejuvenation Institute of Los Angeles (2008) 'Welcome to the Laser Vagina Rejuvenation Institute of Los Angeles'. Online at www.drmatlock.com.

Thomas, B. and Dorling, D. (2007) *Identity in Britain: A Cradle-to-Grave Atlas*. Bristol: Policy Press.

Timmermans, S. (1998) 'Social death as self-fulfilling prophecy: David Sudnow's Passing On revisited'. *The Sociological Quarterly*, 39 (3): 453–472.

—— (2005) 'Death brokering: constructing culturally appropriate deaths'. *Sociology of Health and Illness*, 27 (7): 993, 1013.

—— (2007) *Postmortem: How Medical Examiners Explain Suspicious Deaths* (2nd edn). Chicago, IL: University of Chicago Press.

Townsend, P., Davidson, N. and Whitehead, M. (1992) *Inequalities in Health: The Black Report, The Health Divide* (2nd edn). Harmondsworth: Penguin.

Tozer, J. (2005) 'Hospital blunders "kill 34,000 a year"'. *Daily Mail*, 3 November.

Trottal, F., Apolone, G., Garattini, S. and Tafuri, G. (2008) 'Stopping a trial early in oncology: for patients or for industry?'. *Annals of Oncology*, 9 April. Online at http://annonc.oxfordjournals.org/cgi.

Turner, B. S. (1986) 'The vocabulary of complaints: nursing, professionalism and job context'. *Journal of Sociology*, 22 (3): 368–386.

United Nations (2008) *Human Development Report 2007/2008*. New York: United Nations Development Programme.

United Nations Children's Fund (2008) *The State of the World's Children 2008 Report* (Executive summary). New York: United Nations.

van der Zee, B. (2008) *Rebel, Rebel – The Protestor's Handbbook*. Manchester: Guardian Newspapers.

Wahlberg, K. (2008) 'Are we approaching a global food crisis? Between soaring food prices and food aid shortage'. *Global Policy Forum*. 3 March. Online at www.globalpolicy.org.

Walter, T. (1991) 'Modern death: taboo or not taboo?' *Sociology*, 25 (2): 293–310.

Weber, M. (1948) *From Max Weber: Essays in Sociology* (trans. and eds H. H. Gerth and C. W. Mills). London: Routledge & Kegan Paul.

West, P. (2004) 'The philosopher as dangerous liar'. *New Statesman*, 28 June, 133 (4694): 24–25.

Wicks, D. (1999) *Nurses and Doctors at Work: Rethinking Professional Boundaries*. Sydney: Allen & Unwin.

Wilkinson, A. (1997) 'Sorry state in the States'. *The Guardian*, 12 August.

Wilkinson, G., McKenzie, K. and Harpham, T. (eds) (2005) *Social Capital and Mental Health*. London: Jessica Kingsley.

Wilkinson, I. (2005) *Suffering: A Sociological Introduction*. Cambridge: Polity Press.

Wilkinson, R. (1999) 'Putting the picture together: prosperity, redistribution, health, and welfare'. In M. Marmot and R. G. Wilkinson (eds) *Social Determinants of Health*. Oxford: Oxford University Press, pp. 256–274.

—— (2005) *The Impact of Inequality: How to Make Sick Societies Healthier*. London: Routledge.

—— (2006) *The Impact of Inequality: How to Make Sick Societies Healthier*. New York: New Press.

Williamson, L., Dodds, J., Mercey, D., Hart, G. and Johnson, A. (2008). 'Sexual risk behaviour and knowledge of HIV status among community samples of gay men in the UK'. *AIDS*, 22 (9): 1063–1070.

Wilson, H. and McAndrew, S. (2000) *Sexual Health: Foundations for Practice*. Edinburgh: Bailliere Tindall.

Windsor, C., Prince of Wales (2005) 'Christopher Smallwood's Report on Integrated Health'. 15 October. Online at www.princeofwales.gov.uk/media centre/pressreleases/christopher_smallwood_s_report_on_integrated_health _180.html.

World Bank (2008a) 'World Bank leader says high food prices likely to persist for several years'. 8 April. Online at http://web.worldbank.org.

—— (2008b) 'Financial crisis: what the World Bank is doing'. Online at www. worldbank.org/html/extdr/financial-crisis.

World Health Organization (1946) *Constitution of the World Health Organisation*. Geneva: WHO.

—— (1978) *Alma-Ata 1977*. Copenhagen: WHO.

—— (2005) 'World Health Organization partners with Joint Commission and Joint Commission International to eliminate medical errors worldwide'. Online at www.jointcommissioninternational.org/23194.

—— (2007) *WHO Calls for Prevention of Cancer through Healthy Workplaces*. Geneva: World Health Organization.

—— (2008a) 'Obesity and overweight – facts'. Online at www.who.int.

—— (2008b) 'Mental Health: the bare facts'. Online at www.who.int/mental_health.

—— (2008c) 'Global summary of the HIV and AIDS epidemic, 2006'. Online at www.who.int/globalatlas.

—— (2008d) 'Cancer'. Online at www.who.int/cancer/en.

—— (2008e). 'Why do so many women still die in pregnancy or childbirth?'. Online at www.who.int.

World Wildlife Fund (2008) 'Living Planet Report 2008'. http://assets.panda.org/downloads/living_planet_report_2008.pdf.

Wray, R. (2006) 'First Chinese medicine firm floats in London to fund research. *The Guardian*, 10 April.

Wurtzel, E. (1994) *Prozac Nation: Young and Depressed in America – A Memoir*. New York: Riverhead.

Young, M. and Cullen, L. (1996) *A Good Death*. London: Routledge.

Žižek, S. (2008) *Violence*. London: Profile.

INDEX